Clinical Pocket Manual™

Respiratory Care

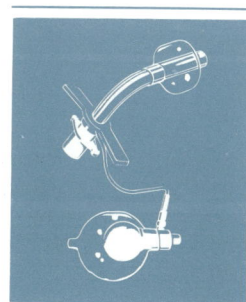

NURSING86 BOOKS™
SPRINGHOUSE CORPORATION
SPRINGHOUSE, PENNSYLVANIA

Clinical Pocket Manual™ Series

PROGRAM DIRECTOR
Jean Robinson

CLINICAL DIRECTOR
Barbara McVan, RN

ART DIRECTOR
John Hubbard

EDITORIAL MANAGER
Susan R. Williams

EDITORS
**Lisa Z. Cohen
Kathy E. Goldberg
Virginia P. Peck**

CLINICAL EDITORS
**Donna Hilton, RN, CCRN, CEN
Joan E. Mason, RN, EdM
Diane Schweisguth, RN, BSN**

COPY SUPERVISOR
David R. Moreau

DESIGNER
Maria Errico

PRODUCTION COORDINATOR
Susan Powell-Mishler

Material in this book was adapted from the following series: Nurse's Reference Library, Nursing Photobook, New Nursing Skillbook, Nursing Now, and Nurse's Clinical Library.

Amended reprint, 1986

CPM6-020586

Library of Congress Cataloging-in-Publication Data

Main entry under title:

Respiratory care.

(Clinical pocket manual)
"Nursing85 books."
Includes index.
1. Respiratory disease nursing—Handbooks, manuals, etc.   I. Series. [DNLM: 1. Respiration Disorders—nursing. WY 163 R4332]
RC735.5.R464 1985   616.2   85-17364
ISBN 0-87434-008-X

CONTENTS

Nursing86 Books™

CLINICAL POCKET MANUAL™ SERIES
Diagnostic Tests
Emergency Care
Fluids and Electrolytes
Signs and Symptoms
Cardiovascular Care
Respiratory Care
Critical Care
Neurologic Care
Surgical Care

NURSING NOW™ SERIES
Shock
Hypertension
Drug Interactions
Cardiac Crises
Respiratory Emergencies
Pain

NURSE'S CLINICAL LIBRARY™
Cardiovascular Disorders
Respiratory Disorders
Endocrine Disorders
Neurologic Disorders
Renal and Urologic Disorders
Gastrointestinal Disorders
Neoplastic Disorders
Immune Disorders

NURSING PHOTOBOOK™ SERIES
Providing Respiratory Care
Managing I.V. Therapy
Dealing with Emergencies
Giving Medications
Assessing Your Patients
Using Monitors
Providing Early Mobility
Giving Cardiac Care
Performing GI Procedures
Implementing Urologic Procedures
Controlling Infection
Ensuring Intensive Care
Coping with Neurologic Disorders
Caring for Surgical Patients
Working with Orthopedic Patients
Nursing Pediatric Patients
Helping Geriatric Patients
Attending Ob/Gyn Patients
Aiding Ambulatory Patients
Carrying Out Special Procedures

NURSE'S REFERENCE LIBRARY®
Diseases
Diagnostics
Drugs
Assessment
Procedures
Definitions
Practices
Emergencies
Signs and Symptoms

NURSE REVIEW™ SERIES
Cardiac Problems
Respiratory Problems
Gastrointestinal Problems
Neurologic Problems
Vascular Problems

Nursing86 DRUG HANDBOOK™

When to Assess the Respiratory System

Respiratory assessment is essential on hospital admission, at regular intervals during illness, and during routine health evaluation and screening. Perform respiratory assessment daily for ambulatory patients and more frequently for patients who are acutely ill or particularly susceptible to disease (pediatric and geriatric patients, for example) or those whose activities are limited by medication, surgery, or debilitating diseases. Your assessment can be deliberate and organized—as it would be for a newly admitted patient. Or it may be informal: For example, during your patient's bath, meals, and ambulation, you may observe for changes in his skin color and in the rate and depth of his respirations, for his use of accessory muscles, and for increased temperature. But whether your assessment is planned or informal, you'll probably be the first person your patient comes in contact with who can detect early changes in his pulmonary function, thus ensuring prompt treatment.

The two vital functions of the respiratory system are maintenance of oxygen and carbon dioxide exchange in the lungs and tissues, and regulation of acid-base balance. Any changes in this system affect all the other body systems. In chronic respiratory disease, changes in pulmonary status (such as hypoxemia) occur slowly, and the person's body has time to adapt. But with acute pulmonary changes, such as those from pneumothorax or aspiration pneumonia, the other body systems don't have time to adapt to sudden hypoxemia, which can cause death.

Changes in other body systems may reduce the lungs' capability to give oxygen. For example, a patient's poor cardiac function results in decreased tissue oxygenation, which causes his lungs to work harder to give oxygen. In fact, any acute disease state increases the body's oxygen demands and the lungs' workload. Also, debilitation from acute disease makes a patient more susceptible to secondary infections, which may affect his lungs.

ASSESSING THE PATIENT

Inspecting the Patient

To properly inspect a patient with a respiratory disorder, look at everything, including his behavior. Examine your patient from head to toe, and document your initial findings on his chart.

HEAD AND NECK

Mental state

• Delirium, confusion, or hallucinations: may mean hypercapnia or severe hypoxemia. (With elderly patients, don't attribute disorientation to age.)

• Fearfulness: seen in patients with acute respiratory distress. They're usually restless, with an anxious expression.

Color

• Pallor: may indicate anemia or hypotension.

• Flushing: may mean patient is retaining carbon dioxide.

• Cyanosis of the buccal mucosa and lips: may indicate hypoxemia, although anemia, if present, may interfere with recognition. Peripheral cyanosis may indicate vascular changes. (If patient has dark skin, check soles of his feet and palms of his hands for duskiness.)

• Pink skin: seen in patients with pure emphysema. Patient usually thin, with cardiac enlargement and sparse sputum production.

• Ruddy skin with blue overtones: seen in patients with pure chronic bronchitis. Patient usually heavyset, with ankle edema and distended neck veins.

Eyes

• Engorged veins, swollen optic discs, or papilledema: may mean patient is retaining carbon dioxide.

Lips

• Pursed lips: seen in patients with COPD. Breathing out through pursed lips helps the patient get rid of more carbon dioxide.

• Circumoral cyanosis (a bluish or dusky ring circling the mouth): may mean the patient has hypoxemia.

Nose

• Nasal flaring: may mean respiratory distress, specifically in infants. May be accompanied by expiratory grunt.

• Nasal polyps: may interfere with respirations.

• Red, swollen nose: may mean allergies.

Neck

• Retraction of accessory muscles: may indicate respiratory distress, especially in patients with COPD.

• Vein engorgement: may suggest high venous pressure.

• Trachea position: should be equidistant from heads of clavicles. With tension pneumothorax or large pleural effusion, trachea will shift *away* from involved side. With atelectasis, trachea may shift *toward* affected side.

Continued

Inspecting the Patient
Continued

CHEST

General observations
● Scars: may mean patient's had surgery.
● Anterior-posterior diameter of chest: should be smaller than the lateral diameter. *Remember:* Chest tends to become barrel-shaped with chronic lung disease.
● Sternum: should be located midline anterior, giving rise to a visible projection known as the Angle of Louis.

Chest movement
● Inspiratory intercostal retractions: occur in patients with COPD, asthma, or pulmonary fibrosis. *Note:* Sudden, violent intercostal and neck retractions can be caused by airway obstruction; for example, aspiration of foreign body.
● Inspiratory intercostal bulges: may mean aneurysm, tumor, or cardiac enlargement.
● Use of accessory muscles during respiration: suggests respiratory distress. Seen in patients with COPD and asthma.
● Localized expiratory bulging: commonly associated with flail chest.
● Abdominal breathing: seen in patients with COPD. During exhalation, patient must retract abdominal muscles to force trapped air from alveoli. This is the patient's unknowing attempt to use his diaphragm to breathe. Teach him the correct way to do diaphragmatic breathing.

Sternal abnormalities
If severe, any of the following can inhibit respiration and ventilation:
● Pigeon chest: associated with rickets or emphysema. In this condition, a softening of the ribs causes the sternum to protrude anteriorly.
● Barrel chest: occurs with emphysema or asthma. Anterior-posterior dimension of the chest enlarges. The ribs tend to be more horizontal than sloped. No bulges. No depression.
● Funnel chest: seen in rickets. Softening of the ribs causes depression of lower sternum.

Spinal abnormalities
If any of the following abnormalities are severe, they can inhibit the patient's respirations and decrease ventilation to his lungs. In some cases, the condition may be obvious. In others, the doctor may need to order an X-ray to determine the diagnosis.
● Kyphosis: Patients with this condition display an abnormally increased convexity of spine.
● Scoliosis: Patients with this condition display a lateral deviation of spine, which results in an S-shaped curve. On concave side of
Continued

Inspecting the Patient
Continued

CHEST
Continued

chest, the patient's ribs are close together. On convex side of chest, his ribs are further apart.
- Kyphoscoliosis: This condition is a combination of kyphosis and scoliosis. The patient's spine is convex, as seen in kyphosis, but it's also S-shaped, as seen in scoliosis.

EXTREMITIES

Skin
- Elevated temperature: suggests infection.
- Diaphoresis or clamminess: may mean hypoxemia or decreased blood pressure.
- Lack of turgor: indicates dehydration.

Fingers and toes
- Clubbing: associated with patients who have COPD, tuberculosis, or chronic hypoxemia. *Remember:* Clubbing's divided into three stages—normal, early, and late. In early clubbing, the angle between the nail and the nail bed is flattened to 180°. In late clubbing, the angle where the nail meets the finger is inverted to 120°.
- Asterixis: To check, pull patient's hand back toward his elbow. Flapping of the middle finger will occur in patients with carbon dioxide narcosis or hepatic failure.

- Nail bed cyanosis: This condition suggests hypoxemia, particularly if it accompanies central cyanosis.

Legs
If your patient displays any of the following conditions, be sure you ask if he's had any previous circulatory problems. Record this history in your notes.
- Thrombophlebitis: This condition may lead to pulmonary emboli. Check the patient's calves for redness, swelling, warmth, and Homans' sign.
- Homans' sign: may mean deep vein thrombosis. To check for it, seat the patient in a chair. Then forcefully dorsiflex his foot. Be sure to document any complaints he has of pain deep in his calf.
- Ankle edema: This condition indicates fluid overload in the patient's body tissues. It may be seen in patients with COPD or right-sided ventricular failure (cor pulmonale). To check for ankle edema, press your fingers into ankle area, hold, and release. Note the impression your fingers leave on his skin. *Remember:* Always document what you've observed in your nurses' notes so it can be used as baseline data. Then anyone who later records changes in the degree of ankle edema will have the data she needs to make an accurate assessment.

Inspecting the Nose, Mouth, and Throat

NOSE

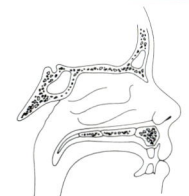

EQUIPMENT
Penlight, nasoscope with light, ophthalmoscope or otoscope with light, or nasal speculum
Procedure
● Observe the size, shape, placement, and general condition of the patient's nose.
Abnormal findings
● Discharge, inflammation, asymmetrical placement
Procedure
● Observe nostrils for symmetry of size and shape.
Abnormal findings
● Flaring nostrils, which suggest respiratory difficulty
Procedure
● Test for nasal obstructions by holding a small mirror under the patient's nostrils. Observe the condensation circles that appear as the patient breathes.
Abnormal findings
● Condensation circles of varying

sizes, indicating a partial nasal obstruction; or an absent condensation circle, indicating total nasal obstruction
Procedure
● Ask the patient to tilt his head back; then, gently push up the tip of his nose. Using a penlight, observe the mucous membranes, septum, and inferior turbinate.
Abnormal findings
● Gray, pale, red, or swollen mucous membranes
● Discharge or purulent drainage
● Foreign object
● Deviated septum (septum that inclines toward one side or the other, giving it an S shape)
● Perforated septum (indicated if light shines through the perforation into opposite nostril)
● Nasal polyps (pale, shiny balls with stalks) attached to turbinate
Procedure
● Using a nasal speculum, carefully expand the nostril and observe the inferior and middle turbinates. *Note:* Don't use a nasal speculum when examining a young or uncooperative child; you may injure him.
Abnormal findings
● Nasal polyps
● Purulent drainage
● Pallor and engorgement (may indicate allergic rhinitis)

Continued

Inspecting the Nose, Mouth, and Throat
Continued

MOUTH AND THROAT

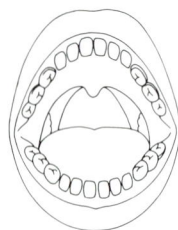

EQUIPMENT
Penlight, tongue depressor
Procedure
● Observe color and condition of lips
Abnormal findings
● Lesions, cyanosis, pallor
  Note: Lips normally are slightly darker than surrounding skin.
Procedure
● Ask the patient to open his mouth and say "Ahh." Observe his mucous membranes. If the patient's Caucasian or Oriental, they should be smooth and pink; if he's black, they should be a patchy pink.
Abnormal findings
● Lesions, bleeding, odor, or tenderness
Procedure
● Observe gums and teeth.
  Nursing tip: Is your patient age

2 or younger? Estimate the number of teeth he should have by subtracting six from the number of months in his age.
Abnormal findings
● Puffy, tender, or bleeding gums
● Discolored, broken, maloccluded teeth; delayed eruption of teeth
  Note: Teach the patient good dental hygiene and refer him to a dentist, if necessary. Also, keep in mind that poor gum condition may indicate malnutrition.
Procedure
● Ask patient to stick out his tongue; observe for velvety-pink appearance.
Abnormal findings
● Smoothness, cracks, coating, glossitis (tongue inflammation), lesions, lack of mobility
Procedure
● Observe palate, uvula, tonsils, and pharynx. *Important:* To avoid stimulating the patient's gag reflex, depress only one side of his tongue at a time.
Abnormal findings
● Cleft palate and/or uvula
● Enlarged, inflamed tonsils
  Note: During childhood, tonsils normally become larger, with a glandular (not smooth) appearance.
● Pus, exudate, or follicles on pharynx

Recognizing Respiratory Patterns

As you're counting your patient's respiratory rate, note his respiratory pattern. Except for an occasional deep breath, is his breathing rhythmical? If his breathing isn't rhythmical, note its depth, rate, and pattern for several minutes. Then document your findings.

This chart will help you recognize the nine major respiratory patterns.

EUPNEA

How to recognize it
Normal respiration rate and rhythm. For adults: 5 to 17 breaths per minute; teenagers: 12 to 20 breaths per minute; children aged 2 to 12: 20 to 30 breaths per minute; newborns: 30 to 50 breaths per minute. Occasional deep breaths at a rate of two to three per minute.

TACHYPNEA

How to recognize it
Increased respiration, as seen in fever, pneumonia, compensatory respiratory alkalosis, respiratory insufficiency, lesions in the brain's respiratory control center, and aspirin poisoning.

BRADYPNEA

How to recognize it
Slower but regular respirations. Can occur when the brain's respiratory control center is affected by opiate narcotics, tumor, alcohol, a metabolic disorder, or respiratory decompensation. Normal during sleep.

APNEA

How to recognize it
Absence of breathing; may be periodic

HYPERPNEA

How to recognize it
Deeper respirations; rate normal

CHEYNE-STOKES

How to recognize it
Respirations gradually become faster and deeper than normal, then slower, over a 30- to 170-second period. Alternating with periods of apnea for 20 to 60 seconds. Causes: increased intracranial pressure, severe congestive heart failure, renal failure, meningitis, and drug overdose.

BIOT'S

How to recognize it
Faster and deeper respirations than normal, with abrupt pauses between them. Each breath has same depth. May occur with spinal meningitis or other CNS conditions.

Continued

Recognizing Respiratory Patterns
Continued

KUSSMAUL'S

How to recognize it
Faster and deeper respirations without pauses. In adults: over 20 breaths per minute. Patient's breathing usually sounds labored, with deep breaths that resemble sighs. Can occur from renal failure or metabolic acidosis, particularly diabetic ketoacidosis.

APNEUSTIC

How to recognize it
Prolonged, gasping inspiration, followed by extremely short, inefficient expiration. Can occur from lesions in the brain's respiratory center.

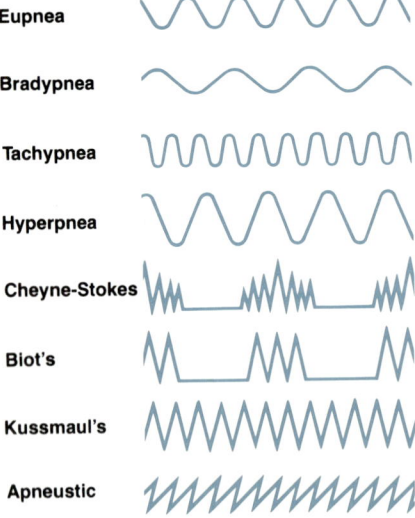

Eupnea

Bradypnea

Tachypnea

Hyperpnea

Cheyne-Stokes

Biot's

Kussmaul's

Apneustic

Identifying Chest Deformities

As you inspect your patient's anterior chest, you may notice deviations in size or shape. The illustrations on pages 9 and 10 demonstrate four such deformities. Note the physical characteristics, signs, and associated conditions typical of each.

FUNNEL CHEST

Physical characteristics
- Sinking or funnel-shaped depression of lower sternum
- Diminished anteroposterior chest diameter

Signs and associated conditions
- Postural disorders, such as forward displacement of neck and shoulders
- Upper thoracic kyphosis
- Protuberant abdomen
- Functional heart murmur

PIGEON CHEST

Physical characteristics
- Projection of sternum beyond abdomen's frontal plane. Evident in two variations: projection greatest at xiphoid process; projection greatest at or near center of sternum

Sign and associated condition
- Functional cardiovascular or respiratory disorders

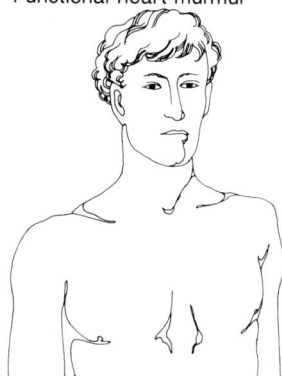

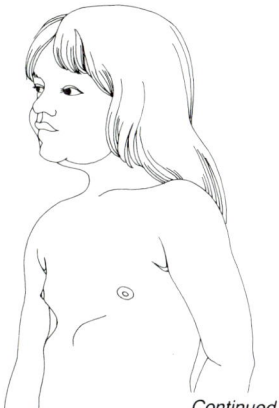

Continued

Identifying Chest Deformities
Continued

BARREL CHEST

Physical characteristics
- Enlarged anteroposterior and transverse chest dimensions; chest appears barrel-shaped
- Prominent accessory muscles

Signs and associated conditions
- Chronic respiratory disorders
- Increasing shortness of breath
- Chronic cough
- Wheezing

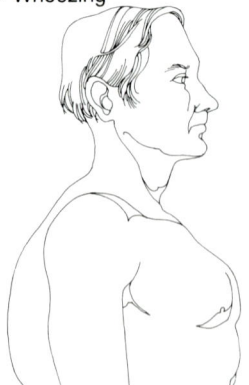

BIFID STERNUM

Physical characteristic
- Complete or incomplete sternal separation

Signs and associated conditions
- Missing or supernumary ribs
- Ectopia cordis (development of heart outside thoracic cavity)

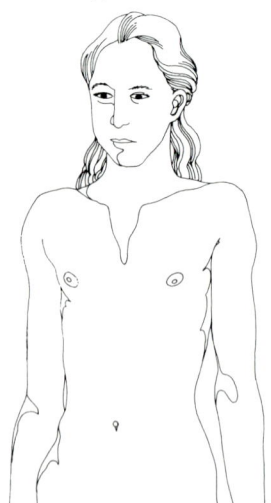

Pediatric Anatomy

While you're examining a child, note any structural abnormalities of his chest. Chest abnormalities in children and their significance include the following:

• An unusually wide space between the nipples may indicate Turner's syndrome. (The distance between the outside areolar edges shouldn't be more than one quarter of the patient's chest circumference.)

• Rachitic beads (bumps at the costochondral junction of the ribs) may indicate rickets.

• Pigeon chest may be a sign of Marfan's or Morquio's syndrome or any chronic upper respiratory tract obstruction; funnel chest may indicate rickets or Marfan's syndrome; barrel chest may indicate chronic respiratory disease, such as cystic fibrosis or asthma.

• Localized bulges may suggest underlying pressures, such as cardiac enlargement or aneurysm.

• Multiple (more than five) café-au-lait spots may be associated with neurofibromatosis.

However, certain *normal* anatomical differences that distinguish a child's respiratory tract make him especially prone to respiratory problems, such as airway obstruction. Here are a few examples:

• A child's mucous membranes are loosely attached to his airway. As a result, they're easily irritated, which may cause edema and coughing.

• His airway is smaller in diameter than an adult's, and contains a greater proportion of soft tissue, including the soft palate and tongue. All of these factors make airway obstruction more likely if excessive mucus formation or edema occurs for any reason.

• An infant's larynx is located two or three cervical vertebrae higher than an adult's, increasing the risk of obstruction by aspiration.

Keep in mind that even an apparently minor respiratory system problem may become life-threatening. When your pediatric patient has such a problem, treat him with special care.

Assessing the Fingers for Clubbing

To quickly assess the fingers for clubbing, have the patient place the first phalanges of the forefingers together. Normally, the bases of the nails are concave and create a small, diamond-shaped space when the first phalanges are opposed (as shown in the top illustration below). When clubbed fingers are opposed, the now convex bases of the nails can touch without leaving a space (as shown in the bottom illustration below).

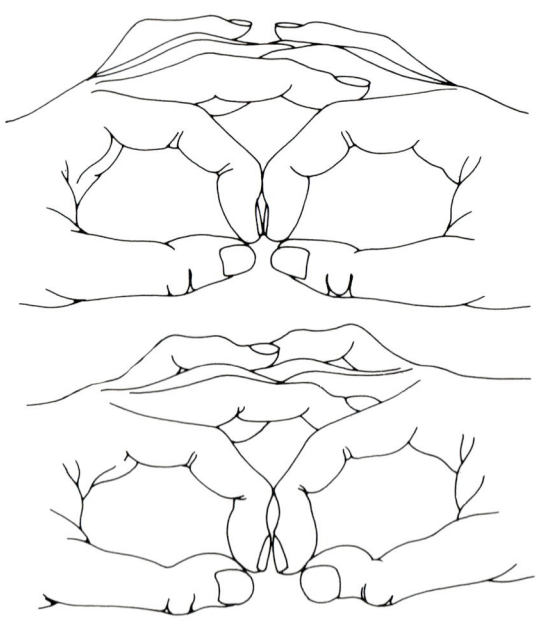

Palpation Sequences

Follow the sequences illustrated here to palpate your patient's posterior and anterior chest.

Posterior

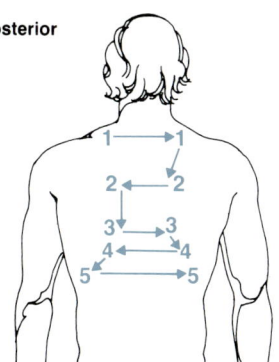

Anterior

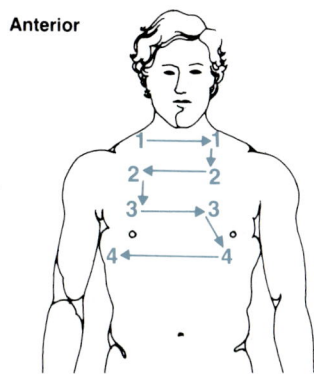

Percussion and Auscultation Sequences

Follow the sequences illustrated here to percuss and auscultate your patient's lungs. Remember to compare sound variations from one side to the other as you pro-ceed, and to avoid bony areas. Document any abnormal sounds and describe them carefully, including their location.

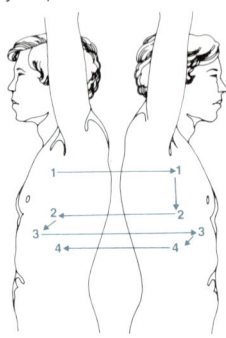

Left lateral   Right lateral

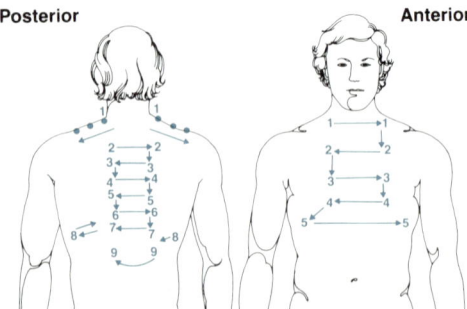

Posterior   Anterior

Guide to Respiratory Sounds

Important: After inspection, lung auscultation is your best assessment tool for most respiratory emergencies. It can detect a bronchial obstruction or air or fluid in the pleural space.

To auscultate, listen with a stethoscope over all lung fields anteriorly, posteriorly, and laterally, if time allows.

Press the stethoscope diaphragm firmly against the patient's skin, wetting his chest hairs if possible to reduce rubbing sounds. Have the patient inhale and exhale slowly and deeply through his mouth.

Compare the sounds on each side of his chest to distinguish normal from adventitious sounds.

Note: If your patient is lying on his side, his uppermost lung will be better ventilated. Keep this in mind when comparing breath sounds.

BRONCHIAL OR TRACHEAL

Pitch
High
Intensity
Loud, predominantly on expiration
Normal findings
When listening over the trachea or mainstem bronchus, you'll hear a sound like air blown through a hollow tube.
Abnormal findings
When you hear bronchial sounds over peripheral lung, it may indicate atelectasis or consolidation.

BRONCHOVESICULAR

Pitch
Moderate
Intensity
Moderate
Normal findings
When listening over large airways, over either side of sternum, Angle of Louis, and between the scapu-

lae, you'll hear a blowing sound.
Abnormal findings
When you hear bronchovesicular sound over peripheral lung, it may indicate consolidation.

VESICULAR

Pitch
High on inspiration; low on expiration
Intensity
Loud on inspiration; soft on expiration
Normal findings
When listening over peripheral lung, you'll hear sounds that have a soft, breezy quality.
Abnormal findings
Decreased sounds in affected peripheral lung may indicate early pneumonia or emphysema. Sounds are decreased because patient's barrel chest causes lungs to be farther from chest wall.

Guide to Adventitious Sounds

Adventitious sounds are abnormal; during auscultation, you may hear them superimposed over your patient's breath sounds. Learn to recognize these sounds and what they tell you about the patient's condition.

CRACKLES—FINE-TO-MEDIUM
(crackles, late inspiratory)

Cause:
Air passing through fluid in small air passages and alveoli
Description:
Noncontinuous crackling sounds. (To simulate, rub a few hairs together over your ear.) Heard at end of inspiration, over the peripheral lung. If widespread, usually indicates pneumonia. Also found in congestive heart failure.

CRACKLES—MEDIUM-TO-COARSE
(crackles, early inspiratory)

Cause:
Air passing through fluid in the bronchioles, bronchi, and trachea
Description:
Louder than fine rales. Usually heard on late inspiration or expiration over airways. Heard in bronchitis, bronchiectasis, resolving pneumonia, emphysema, pleural effusion, and congestive heart failure.

RHONCHI—SIBILANT
(wheeze)

Cause:
Air passing through wet and swollen airways
Description:
Continuous high-pitched wheeze sound heard over airways, more pronounced during exhalation. Found in patients with asthma and chronic obstructive pulmonary disease. *Caution:* Absence in asthmatic patient may indicate acute bronchospasm.

RHONCHI—SONOROUS

Cause:
Same as for sibilant
Description:
Continuous low-pitched moaning sound. May clear with coughing. Heard mainly during exhalation. Indicates secretions or obstruction in the larger airways.

FRICTION OR PLEURAL RUB

Cause:
Rubbing together of inflamed and irritated pleural surfaces
Description:
Grating sound. Heard during inspiration and exhalation. Found in patients with pleurisy, TB, pulmonary infarction, pneumonia, or lung cancer.

How to Percuss Your Patient's Chest

The sounds you hear when you percuss your patient's chest can help to identify and locate any abnormalities in his lungs. Use these guidelines to aid you in mastering this important assessment skill.

NOTE AND LOCATION	PITCH	INTENSITY	QUALITY
Resonance; normal lung	Low	Moderate to loud	Hollow
Hyperresonance; emphysematous lung or pneumo-thorax	Low	Loud	Booming
Tympany; abdomen distended with air	High	Loud	Musical, drum-like
Dullness; liver, pleural effusion	High	Soft	Thudlike
Flatness; sternum, atelectatic lung	High	Soft	Extreme dull-ness

Nursing Tip

Remember that when you use the lateral position to examine your patient's posterior chest, the bed mattress and the organ displacement involved distort sounds and lung expansion. To offset these effects, examine the uppermost side of your patient's chest first; then roll him on his other side and repeat the examination, for comparison.

When you assess the patient's thorax, keep in mind the three thoracic portions to be examined—posterior, anterior, and lateral. You can examine any of these areas first and perform the lateral examination during the posterior or anterior assessment. The most important point is to *proceed systematically*, always comparing one side of the patient's thorax with the other side. (In this way, the patient serves as his own control.) Remember to examine the apices during the posterior and the anterior examinations.

Assessing for Resonance

If you detect any respiratory abnormality during palpation, percussion, or auscultation, assess the patient's voice sounds for vocal resonance. The significance of vocal resonance is based on the principle that sound carries best through a solid, less well through fluid, and poorly through air. Normally, you should hear vocal resonance as muffled, unclear sounds, loudest medially and less intense at the lung periphery. Voice sounds that become louder and more distinct at the lung periphery signal bronchophony, an abnormal finding except over the trachea and posteriorly over the upper right lobe. To elicit bronchophony, ask your patient to say "99" or "one, two, three," while you auscultate the thorax systematically. Bronchophony usually accompanies enhanced fremitus, abnormal bronchial breath sounds, and dullness on percussion.

Check for whispered pectoriloquy, which is an exaggerated form of bronchophony. Ask the patient to whisper a simple phrase like "one, two, three." Normally, whispered words sound faint and indistinct. Hearing the words clearly through the stethoscope is an abnormal finding. Because whispered pectoriloquy precedes bronchophony, it aids early diagnosis of pneumonia.

Egophony is another form of abnormal vocal resonance. Ask the patient to say "ee, ee." Transmission of the sound through the stethoscope as "ay, ay," is an abnormal finding, possibly indicating compressed lung tissue, as in pleural effusion.

You may hear increased vocal resonance, whispered pectoriloquy, and egophony in any patient with consolidated lungs.

Nursing Tip

Before auscultating for breath sounds, teach your patient how to breathe properly. Demonstrate the appropriate technique by standing in front of your patient and breathing slowly and deeply through your mouth. Mouth breathing doesn't interfere with clear auscultation of the thorax.

Analyzing Your Patient's Cough

By interpreting your patient's cough pattern, cough sounds, and sputum, you can learn valuable information about his condition. This chart tells you how. Ask your patient these questions or, if possible, answer them yourself:

QUESTION/ANSWER	POSSIBLE CAUSES
When do you cough?	
• Early morning	• Chronic inflammation of large airways in patients who smoke
• Late afternoon	• Exposure to irritants during the workday
• Evening	• Chronic postnasal drip or sinusitis, gastric reflux with nocturnal aspiration
What does the cough sound like?	
• Dry	• Cardiac condition
• Barking	• Croup or influenza
• Hacking	• Atypical pneumonia or mycoplasmal pneumonia
• Congested	• Cold, pneumonia, bronchitis
If you're coughing up sputum, what does it looks like?	
• Mucoid	• Tracheobronchitis, asthma
• Yellow or green	• Some bacterial infections
• Rust-colored	• Pneumococcal pneumonia, pulmonary infarction, tuberculosis
• Pink and frothy	• Pulmonary edema

ASSESSING THE PATIENT

Assessing Emergency Respiratory Situations

Respiratory assessment of the emergency patient is critical because life-threatening problems may impair oxygen delivery to tissues.

Begin your assessment by simultaneously checking airway patency and adequate ventilation.

- Observe the chest for rise and fall.
- Listen to the sound of air movement near your patient's mouth and nose.
- Feel for air movement over his mouth and nose.

Use this chart to assess the emergency situation properly.

CONDITION/NURSING ASSESSMENT	NURSING INTERVENTION
Acute respiratory arrest • No respiratory movement • No air felt over mouth and nose	• Position airway, using the head-tilt or jaw-thrust method. • Start mouth-to-mouth resuscitation immediately. • Once you've accomplished ventilation, continue until no longer needed. • Use endotracheal intubation and manual (or mechanical) ventilation, as ordered, for long-term support.
Partial airway obstruction • Increased respiratory effort (orthopnea in conscious patients) • Noisy respirations (whistling, wheezing, crowing) • Use of accessory muscles, including abdominals, sternocleidomastoid, and internal intercostals to try to breathe • Possible intercostal retractions along with nasal flaring	• If patient can speak or cough, let patient attempt to relieve obstruction. • If unsuccessful, administer back blows in succession. (This condition is unlikely to be relieved by an abdominal thrust or by chest compression.) • Administer oxygen until direct laryngoscopy becomes available.

Continued

Assessing Emergency Respiratory Situations
Continued

CONDITION/NURSING   NURSING INTERVENTIONS
ASSESSMENT

Complete airway obstruction
• No respiratory movement
• No air felt over mouth and nose
• If conscious, patient attempts to speak but fails, and typically reaches for his throat

• Administer four rapid blows between the scapulae, followed by the abdominal thrust or compression of the midchest, as is done in external cardiac massage.
• If airway remains obstructed, manual clearing may locate and remove obstruction.
• Anticipate cricothyrotomy or tracheotomy if other attempts fail. Perform cricothyrotomy only in life-threatening emergency when a doctor is unavailable. Usually, a doctor performs a tracheotomy in the operating room.

How to Handle a Respiratory Emergency

When your patient suddenly develops a respiratory emergency, remain calm and complete a thorough assessment by taking the following important steps:
• Assess ABCs (airway, breathing, and circulation) immediately.
• Try to determine cause, and take steps to relieve airway obstruction.
• Administer oxygen. However, before you do, consider the patient's *primary* condition. For example, suppose your steroid-dependent asthmatic patient has an acute attack and is in respiratory crisis. He needs corticosteroids to control his bronchial inflammation before you can administer oxygen.
• Call for help. Don't leave the patient alone until his breathing is stable.
• Ask the patient only questions to which he can answer yes or no—to save his breath and your time.
• Take his vital signs and compare them with the baseline vital signs recorded on his chart.
• Perform a brief physical examination, again consulting his chart for baseline information.

Common Lung Conditions: Signs and Symptoms

Suppose you've just performed a chest assessment. The results indicate that your patient has a respiratory problem, but you're not sure which one. Compare his signs and symptoms with those listed in this chart. He may have one of the following common lung conditions.

PNEUMOTHORAX

Inspection
Dyspnea; less motion on affected side. Trachea may deviate away from affected side.
Palpation
Decreased fremitus
Percussion
Hyperresonance
Auscultation
Decreased or absent breath sounds over affected side

PLEURAL EFFUSION

Inspection
Dyspnea; less-defined intercostal spaces on affected side
Palpation
Decreased fremitus
Percussion
Flatness; decreased diaphragmatic excursion
Auscultation
Decreased or absent breath sounds over involved area

ATELECTASIS

Inspection
Less motion and decreased volume of thorax on affected side. Trachea deviates toward affected side.

Palpation
Varied fremitus
Percussion
Dullness
Auscultation
Transient fine crackles

CONSOLIDATION

Inspection
Less motion on affected side
Palpation
Increased fremitus
Percussion
Dullness to flatness
Auscultation
Medium-to-coarse crackles; transient friction rub

CONGESTIVE HEART FAILURE (CHF) WITHOUT EFFUSIONS

Inspection
Mostly normal
Palpation
Normal
Percussion
Normal
Auscultation
Fine-to-medium crackles, louder on right than left side

Summary of Assessment Findings

CHRONIC BRONCHITIS

History
- Long-term cigarette smoking
- Long-term exposure to air pollutants
- Productive cough (with clear sputum) that worsens in morning
- Gradual onset of shortness of breath

Inspection
- Cyanosis and edema ("blue bloater")
- Digital clubbing (in later stages)
- Tachypnea
- Use of accessory muscles to breathe
- Occasional intercostal retractions
- In advanced stages, patient sits leaning forward, hands on thighs

Auscultation
- Normal breath sounds
- Fine-to-coarse rales; clear after coughing, wheezing, and/or rhonchi
- Prolonged expiration

Percussion
- Dull or flat sounds over areas of mucous plugging
- Resonant sounds
- Decreased diaphragmatic excursion

Palpation
- Normal voice sounds and fremitus
- Decreased diaphragmatic excursion

EMPHYSEMA

History
- Long-term cigarette smoking
- Long-term exposure to air pollutants
- Nonproductive cough
- Progressive shortness of breath leading to dyspnea on exertion
- Recent weight loss

Inspection
- Prolonged, labored expirations, without cyanosis or edema ("pink puffer")
- Use of accessory muscles to breathe
- Digital clubbing (in later stages)
- Decreased chest expansion
- In advanced stages, patient sits leaning forward, hands on thighs

Auscultation
- Decreased breath sounds
- Fine crackles at bases and occasional wheezing or rhonchi
- Prolonged expiration

Percussion
- Hyperresonance
- Decreased diaphragmatic excursion

Palpation
- Decreased vocal and tactile fremitus
- Decreased diaphragmatic excursion

Continued

Summary of Assessment Findings
Continued

CYSTIC FIBROSIS

History
• Family history of cystic fibrosis
• Productive cough (with copious sputum)
• Shortness of breath on exertion
• Weight loss or failure to gain weight
Inspection
• Barrel chest
• Cyanosis
• Digital clubbing
Auscultation
• Fine rales and coarse rhonchi
Percussion
• Hyperresonance
• Dull or flat sounds over areas of mucous plugging
• Decreased diaphragmatic excursion
Palpation
• Decreased vocal and tactile fremitus

BRONCHIECTASIS

History
• Frequent respiratory infections
• History of cystic fibrosis or cancer
• Frequent, productive cough with copious, foul-smelling sputum
• Hemoptysis
Inspection
• Cyanosis
• Dyspnea
• Digital clubbing

Auscultation
• Fine rales and coarse rhonchi
Percussion
• Dull or flat sounds
• Decreased diaphragmatic excursion
Palpation
• Increased vocal and tactile fremitus

ASTHMA

History
• Allergic predisposition
• Exposure to allergen or stress, or ingestion of aspirin or indomethacin
Inspection
• Dyspnea
• Tachypnea
• Intercostal retractions (inspiration) and bulging (expiration)
• Accessory muscles use
• Flaring nostrils
• Cyanosis
• Digital clubbing
Auscultation
• Wheezing and rhonchi
• Unequal breath sounds
• Tachycardia
• Paradoxical pulse
Percussion
• Hyperresonance
• Decreased diaphragmatic excursion
Palpation
• Decreased vocal and tactile fremitus

Forming Sample Nursing Diagnoses

CHIEF COMPLAINT/EFFECT OF SIGN OR SYMPTOM	NURSING DIAGNOSIS
Dyspnea	
Acute:	
• Diaphoresis; restlessness	• Alterations in comfort
Chronic:	
• Barrel chest; accessory muscle change	• Ineffective breathing pattern
Acute and chronic:	
• Fatigue, exhaustion	• Fear of breathlessness, ineffective breathing pattern, impaired gas exchange, impaired physical mobility
• Emotional distress	
• Hypoventilation/hyperventilation (may lead to respiratory acidosis/alkalosis)	
Chest pain	
• Decreased ventilation (may lead to infection or increased CO_2 retention and respiratory acidosis)	• Impaired gas exchange, ineffective breathing pattern
• Discomfort	• Fear of chest pain, alterations in comfort
• Pain	
Cough	
Chronic and short-term (less than 1 month):	
• Hazardous elevation in intrathoracic pressure, intracranial pressure, and blood pressure (may lead to congestive heart failure, ruptured aneurysm)	• Impaired gas exchange
• Cough syncope	
• Musculoskeletal pain	• Alterations in comfort
• Fractured ribs	

Continued

Forming Sample Nursing Diagnoses
Continued

CHIEF COMPLAINT/EFFECT OF SIGN OR SYMPTOM	NURSING DIAGNOSIS

Cough
Continued
Chronic and long-term (more than 1 month):
- Fatigue
- Weight loss, anorexia

    • Alteration in nutrition (less than body requirements)

Forced cough:
- Collapsed airways (atelectasis)
- Rupture of thin-walled alveoli (may lead to pneumothorax)
- Hemoptysis, second-degree irritation of tracheobronchial tree

    • Impaired gas exchange

    • Alteration in comfort

Increased and abnormal secretions
Increased sputum:
- Mucous plugs (may lead to airway obstruction, atelectasis, prevention of alveoli gas exchange, hypoxemia, respiratory acidosis)
- Increased secretions and/or abnormal fluids retained in lung (may lead to infection, tracheobronchitis, bronchopneumonia)

    • Ineffective airway clearance, impaired gas exchange

Hemoptysis:
- Obstruction with blood (may lead to asphyxiation, atelectasis, pneumonia)

    • Ineffective airway clearance, impaired gas exchange, alterations in tissue perfusion

- Blood-streaked sputum; severe blood loss may lead to shock

Assessment Questions for COPD

Begin your assessment of the COPD patient with a carefully detailed history. To start with, ask the patient and his family:

• Does he smoke? If so, obtain a smoking history in pack years. (To calculate pack years, multiply the number of packs smoked per day by the number of years the patient's been smoking.)

• Does he cough? Does the cough produce sputum? What does the sputum look like? When did the cough begin? What time of day does it occur? Does it worsen at any particular time?

• Does he ever experience breathlessness?

• Does breathlessness worsen at any time of day or with any particular activity? Does it limit his activities?

• Does he have difficulty breathing when lying down?

• Does the patient's work expose him to respiratory irritants?

• Does his family have a history of allergies?

• Was he exposed recently to a specific allergen, a nonspecific respiratory irritant, or unusual emotional stress?

• Has the patient ever had chronic interstitial pneumonitis or fibrosis, recurrent pulmonary thromboembolism, polycythemia vera, myxedema, or obesity-hyperventilation syndrome?

• Does he suffer from unusual fatigue, anterior chest pain, and palpitations on exertion (all signs of cor pulmonale)?

• Does he suffer from ankle edema, increased epigastric fullness, and upper abdominal aching (possible signs of right ventricular failure)?

COPD Facts

• Habitual cigarette smoking is by far the most common cause of COPD; COPD rarely occurs in nonsmokers.
• Because onset of COPD is often insidious, early diagnosis is rare. Symptoms usually don't occur until the disease is advanced.

• Avoiding bronchopulmonary irritants, especially during exacerbations of respiratory symptoms, is the key to treatment of COPD. The goal of treatment is to help the patient maintain optimal breathing function and activity level rather than to cure the disease.

COPD Assessment Findings

Use this chart to compare the three primary causes of chronic obstructive pulmonary disease (COPD). But remember, assessment findings may vary from one patient to the next, depending on the condition's severity and the presence or absence of complications.

CHRONIC BRONCHITIS

Onset
Insidious; usually affects patients over age 40 who smoke
Signs and symptoms
• Chronic, productive cough that's worse in the mornings and during cold weather
• Exertional dyspnea
• Use of accessory muscles for breathing

• Rhonchi and wheezes on auscultation
History
• Long-term smoking
• Chronic cough for at least 3 months a year for two successive years
• Recurrent episodes of diaphoresis (especially at night)
• Recurrent respiratory tract infections

Continued

COPD Assessment Findings
Continued

CHRONIC BRONCHITIS
Continued

Diagnostic test results
● Chest X-ray: may show hyperinflation and increased bronchovascular markings
● Pulmonary function tests: normal in early stage; as condition progresses, tests show increased residual volume, decreased vital capacity and forced expiratory volumes, normal static compliance and diffusing capacity
● Decreased PaO_2, normal or elevated $PaCO_2$
● Sputum: thick; grey, yellow, or white; contains microorganisms and neutrophils
● EKG: may show atrial dysrhythmias; peaked P waves in leads II, III, and aVF; and possibly right ventricular hypertrophy
● Complete blood count: elevated leukocytes if a bacterial infection's present

EMPHYSEMA

Onset
Insidious; most often affects patients over age 60

Signs and symptoms
● Exertional dyspnea
● Chronic but relatively unproductive cough
● Weight loss
● Prolonged expiratory period with grunting, pursed-lip breathing, tachypnea
● Use of accessory muscles to breathe
● Hyperresonance on percussion, increased breath sounds, quiet heart sounds
● Anorexia and malaise
● Barrel chest
● Peripheral cyanosis and digital clubbing
History
● Chronic cough and exertional dyspnea for 5 years or more
● Long-term smoker and/or history of bronchitis
● Recurrent respiratory tract infections
● Family history of asthma or alpha₁-antitrypsin deficiency
Diagnostic test results
● Chest X-ray: in moderate to advanced disease, flattened diaphragm, reduced vascular markings at lung periphery,

Continued

COPD Assessment Findings
Continued

EMPHYSEMA
Continued

over-aeration of lungs, vertical heart, enlarged antero-posterior chest diameter, large retrosternal air space
• Pulmonary function tests: in moderate to advanced disease, increased total lung capacity and residual volume, decreased vital capacity and forced expiratory volumes, increased static compliance and decreased expiratory volumes
• Decreased PaO_2; normal $PaCO_2$ (until late in the disease)
• EKG: tall, symmetric P waves in leads II, III, and aVF; vertical QRS axis; signs of right ventricular hypertrophy late in disease
• Increased hemoglobin late in disease when persistent severe hypoxemia develops

ASTHMA

Onset
Childhood onset associated with allergy; adult onset may be unrelated to allergy

Signs and symptoms
During an attack:
• Mild-to-severe dyspnea and wheezing; chest tightness
• Productive cough (clear, white or yellow, tenacious mucus)
• Hyperinflated chest; use of accessory muscles to breathe
• Flared nostrils
• Anxiety; diaphoresis
• Tachycardia, hypertension, pulsus paradoxus
• On auscultation, rhonchi and wheezing throughout lung fields on expiration and possibly inspiration; absent or diminished breath sounds during severe obstruction. Unequal intensity of breath sounds reflects uneven air distribution in the lungs. Bilateral wheezing may be audible without a stethoscope.
Between attacks:
• Patient may be asymptomatic
• Chronic sustained attacks may lead to smooth muscle hypertrophy and may narrow the respiratory tract; patient may then develop chronic symptoms similar to those
Continued

COPD Assessment Findings
Continued

ASTHMA
Continued

caused by chronic bronchitis and emphysema
History
• Intermittent attacks of dyspnea and wheezing; may occur most often at night, after exposure to certain allergens, or during periods of emotional stress
• Eczema, urticaria, seasonal or other allergies (including allergies to aspirin or other drugs), sinus problems, colds and other respiratory infections, or nasal polyps
Diagnostic test results
During an attack:
• Chest X-ray: hyperinflated lungs with air trapping; areas of atelectasis possible
• Sputum: presence of Curschmann's spirals (airway casts), eosinophils, and Charcot-Leyden crystals (breakdown products from eosinophils)
• Pulmonary function tests: decreased forced expiratory volume that improves significantly after administration of inhalation bronchodilator; increased residual volume and functional residual capacity; total lung capacity may also increase
• ABGs: decreased PaO_2; $PaCO_2$ values variable. *Caution:* Rising $PaCO_2$ levels and decreasing pH indicate acidosis and impending respiratory failure
• EKG: sinus tachycardia; during severe attack, signs of cor pulmonale (right axis deviation, peaked P wave) may appear

Nursing Tip

Never administer a high percentage of oxygen to a patient with chronic asthma or another form of COPD. If you do, he may stop breathing. Here's why: A normal person breathes because his respiratory system's stimulated by an increased $PaCO_2$ level. But a COPD patient may consistently retain a high level of carbon dioxide from hypoventilation. Over time, his respiratory center compensates, no longer responding to increased $PaCO_2$ levels. Hypoxemia then becomes his only breathing stimulus. Administering oxygen at a high percentage could depress his hypoxic drive and may lead to respiratory arrest.

How Anxiety Affects Assessment Findings

Anxiety is characteristic when the patient fears breathlessness or pleuritic pain. Because anxiety can change or even obscure assessment findings, it's important to evaluate the patient's level of anxiety first. Is the patient too anxious to respond appropriately to your questions? Is pain or dyspnea increasing his anxiety? Is the patient's family contributing to or reducing anxiety?

Remember that a thorough patient interview and physical examination may only heighten the patient's anxiety, thereby increasing the work of breathing and oxygen consumption. Consequently, do not attempt a complete admission assessment for the patient with obvious distress. Instead, restrict the initial interview to a few "yes or no" questions. And aim to reduce the patient's anxiety by asking questions like "Where is the chest pain?" or "Do you always have trouble breathing, or only when you lie down?" Obtain additional information from the patient's family if possible. Otherwise, wait to complete the assessment. Continue the interview and physical examination after the patient receives oxygen and pain medication and has rested for at least 8, but preferably 24, hours.

Because anxiety can affect assessment findings, evaluate the patient's level of anxiety before performing a complete physical examination. Watch for these signs.

Appearance
- Muscular tension (rigidity)
- Pale, clammy skin
- Fatigue
- Increased small motor activity (restlessness)

Conversation
- Asks many questions
- Shifts topic of conversation
- Describes fears with sense of helplessness
- Avoids focusing on feelings

Behavior
- Shortened attention span
- Inability to follow directions
- Increased acting out

Physiologic signs
- Increased heart and respiratory rate
- Extreme shifts in body temperature, blood pressure, and menstrual flow
- Diarrhea, urinary urgency
- Loss of appetite
- Increased perspiration
- Dilation of pupils

Evaluating Respiratory Status

TEST	PURPOSE

Volumetric tests
Lung capacity
  Vital capacity
  Inspiratory capacity
  Functional residual capacity
  Total lung capacity
  Forced vital capacity
  Forced expiratory volume
  Maximal midexpiratory flow
  Maximal breathing capacity
  Maximal voluntary ventilation
	Assess function
	● Evaluates ventilatory function of lungs; screens for pulmonary disorders
	● Helps classify pulmonary disorders as restrictive or obstructive
	● Evaluates severity of any pulmonary disorder

Lung volume
  Tidal volume
  Minute volume
  Inspiratory reserve volume
  Expiratory reserve volume
  Residual volume
	● Evaluates ventilatory function of lungs; screens for pulmonary disorders
	● Helps classify pulmonary disorders as restrictive or obstructive
	● Evaluates severity of any pulmonary disorder

Visualization tests Bronchoscopy Mediastinoscopy	*Assess structure* ● Directly examines larger airways of tracheobronchial tree ● Directly examines mediastinum for biopsy (usually supplements bronchoscopy)
Radiographic tests Chest radiography Lung scan	*Assess structure, function, and vascular status* ● Visualizes appearance of lungs and helps assess pulmonary status ● Visualizes distribution of blood flow patterns in lungs

Continued

Evaluating Respiratory Status
Continued

TEST	PURPOSE
Radiographic tests *Continued*	**Assess structure, function, and vascular status**
Ventilation scan	• Evaluates ventilatory function
Fluoroscopy	• Visualizes thoracic organs in motion
Tomography	• Supplements radiographs; visualizes target areas in a series of planes to reveal occult pathology
Thoracic computerized tomography	• Locates suspected neoplasms
Bronchography	• Visualizes size and appearance of tracheobronchial tree
Pulmonary angiography	• Visualizes pulmonary vascular system

Respiratory Crisis: Testing Priorities

If your patient's in respiratory crisis, the doctor will order any or all of the following diagnostic tests.
Arterial blood gas (ABG) analysis. Expect the doctor to order ABG measurements immediately since this test requires only a blood specimen yet provides crucial diagnostic information. Although a specially trained nurse may perform the test, you may be responsible for interpreting ABG measurements.
Pulmonary function tests. In most cases, you'll wait until the patient's airway is stable before calling a respiratory therapist to perform appropriate pulmonary function tests. However, you may need to measure the patient's vital capacity and tidal volume without waiting.
Thoracentesis. If the doctor suspects pleural effusion, he may order thoracentesis. (He may also perform this procedure to relieve increased intrapleural pressure.)
Chest X-rays. If a portable X-ray machine's available, the doctor may order chest X-rays immediately. Assist the technician by positioning the patient.

Allen's Test . . . First

Your patient needs an arterial line or arterial blood gas measurement *now*. Despite the urgency, do the Allen's test first. Why? Because these procedures invade the radial artery and may damage it. Since the hand's only other main blood source is the ulnar artery, you need to make sure that's patent *before* the procedure. Here's how:
• Have your patient clench his fist. Next, compress his radial and ulnar arteries.
• Have him unclench his fist. His palm will blanch because you're stopping the blood flow.
• Release pressure from the ulnar artery *only*. If blood flow's adequate, his palm will flush within 5 seconds. If blood flow's inadequate, you'll have to find another insertion site.

Drawing Arterial Blood for Blood Gas Measurements: Some Special Tips

When drawing arterial blood for blood gas measurements, *don't numb the area with a local anesthetic like xylocaine.* First, it will delay the procedure unnecessarily. Second, the patient may have an allergic reaction to the drug. Third, the vasoconstriction produced by the drug may keep you from doing a successful puncture.
• Prepare the needle and ice out of the patient's sight. Speak softly and calmly, reassuring him as much as possible. Take extra time locating the artery so you're successful with the first puncture.
• *Don't turn off any oxygen the patient's receiving*, unless ordered. But check the patient's chart to make sure he's been getting the prescribed oxygen concentration for at least 15 minutes before you draw the blood. Indicate the liter flow on the slip you send to the lab. If no oxygen's in use, simply indicate that the patient's breathing room air (21% oxygen).
• *If the patient's just had an IPPB treatment, wait approximately 20 minutes before drawing arterial blood.* Any less could alter the blood gas measurement.

Understanding ABGs

Arterial blood gas (ABG) analysis evaluates gas exchange in the lungs by measuring the partial pressures of oxygen (PaO_2) and carbon dioxide ($PaCO_2$) and the pH of an arterial sample. PaO_2 indicates how much oxygen the lungs are delivering to the blood. $PaCO_2$ indicates how effi-

	NORMAL	RESPIRATORY ACIDOSIS
Possible causes		Impaired alveolar ventilation, respiratory depressants, intracranial tumors
Symptoms		Lethargy; shallow, irregular respirations; disorientation
Signs		Hypoventilation, asterixis
pH	7.35 to 7.45	Decreased
PaO_2	80 to 100 mm Hg	Normal or decreased
$PaCO_2$	35 to 45 mm Hg	Increased
HCO_3^-	22 to 26 mEq/liter	Increased (compensating)
RR*	10 to 20/min	Decreased

*Respiratory rate

ASSESSING THE PATIENT

Understanding ABGs

ciently the lungs eliminate carbon dioxide. The pH indicates the acid-base level of the blood, or the hydrogen ion (H^+) concentration. Acidity indicates H^+ excess; alkalinity, H^+ deficit. Use the chart below as a guide when interpreting a patient's ABG findings.

RESPIRATORY ALKALOSIS	METABOLIC ACIDOSIS	METABOLIC ALKALOSIS
Ventilatory support, hyperventilation, CNS disease, anxiety, persistent fever, liver disease, CHF, pulmonary embolism	Aspirin, renal disease, diabetes, lactic acidosis, diarrhea, biliary fistulae	Vomiting, diuretics, hyperadrenocorticism, alkali ingestion, hyperaldosteronism, nasogastric suction
Hyperactive reflexes, blurred vision, tetany, vertigo, muscle cramps, sighing, diaphoresis, paresthesias	Kussmaul's respiration, restlessness, disorientation	Weakness, paralysis, leg cramps, paresthesias
Hyperventilation, latent tetany	Shock, coma, tachypnea	Hypokalemic symptoms (nausea, weakness)
Increased	Decreased	Increased
Normal or increased	Normal or increased	Normal or decreased
Decreased	Decreased (compensating)	Increased (compensating)
Decreased (compensating)	Decreased	Increased
Increased	Increased (compensating)	Decreased (compensating)

How Respiratory Disorders Affect ABGs

Below is a chart that shows you normal ABG values and how respiratory disorders affect them.

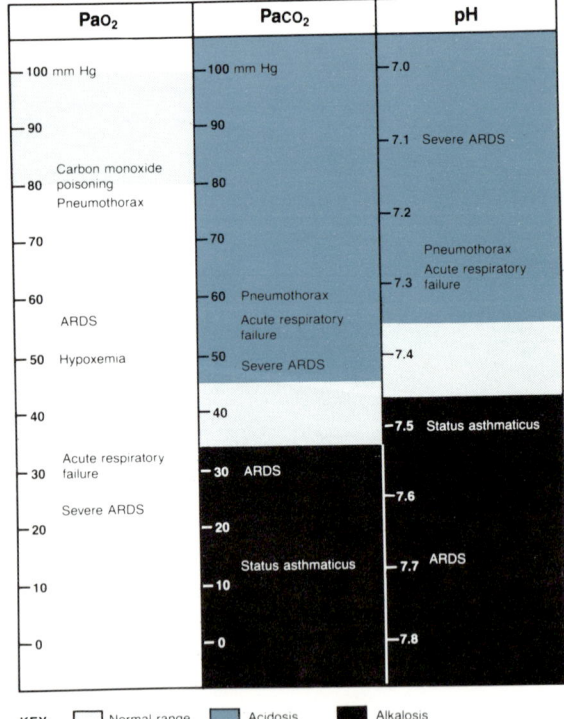

PaO$_2$	PaCO$_2$	pH
— 100 mm Hg	— 100 mm Hg	— 7.0
— 90	— 90	
		— 7.1 Severe ARDS
— 80 Carbon monoxide poisoning Pneumothorax	— 80	
		— 7.2
— 70	— 70	
		Pneumothorax
		Acute respiratory
— 60	— 60 Pneumothorax	— 7.3 failure
ARDS	Acute respiratory failure	
— 50 Hypoxemia	— 50 Severe ARDS	— 7.4
— 40	— 40	— 7.5 Status asthmaticus
— 30 Acute respiratory failure	— 30 ARDS	— 7.6
Severe ARDS		
— 20	— 20	— 7.7 ARDS
	Status asthmaticus	
— 10	— 10	
— 0	— 0	— 7.8

KEY: ☐ Normal range   ▣ Acidosis   ■ Alkalosis

Evaluating Acid-Base Compensation

Is your patient's system attempting to compensate for an acid-base imbalance? Use this diagram to find out. When blood pH reveals alkalemia or acidemia and the primary imbalance is respiratory (resulting from an abnormal $PaCO_2$ level), check the HCO_3^-

If the HCO_3^- level also is abnormal, compensation is occurring. Or, if the primary imbalance is metabolic (resulting from an abnormal HCO_3^- level), check the $PaCO_2$ level. An abnormal $PaCO_2$ level indicates compensation.

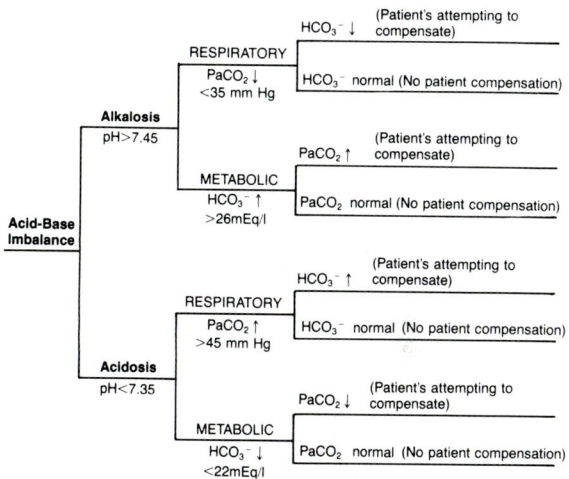

Acid-Base Imbalance

Alkalosis pH>7.45

RESPIRATORY $PaCO_2 \downarrow$ <35 mm Hg
- $HCO_3^- \downarrow$ (Patient's attempting to compensate)
- HCO_3^- normal (No patient compensation)

METABOLIC $HCO_3^- \uparrow$ >26mEq/l
- $PaCO_2 \uparrow$ (Patient's attempting to compensate)
- $PaCO_2$ normal (No patient compensation)

Acidosis pH<7.35

RESPIRATORY $PaCO_2 \uparrow$ >45 mm Hg
- $HCO_3^- \uparrow$ (Patient's attempting to compensate)
- HCO_3^- normal (No patient compensation)

METABOLIC $HCO_3^- \downarrow$ <22mEq/l
- $PaCO_2 \downarrow$ (Patient's attempting to compensate)
- $PaCO_2$ normal (No patient compensation)

ASSESSING THE PATIENT

Interpreting Pulmonary Function Tests

MEASUREMENT OF PULMONARY FUNCTION	METHOD OF CALCULATION	IMPLICATIONS
Tidal volume (V_T) (amount of air inhaled or exhaled during normal breathing)	Determine the spirographic measurement for 10 breaths divided by 10.	Decreased V_T may indicate restrictive disease and requires further testing, such as full pulmonary function study or chest radiography.
Minute volume (V_E) (total amount of air breathed per minute)	Multiply V_T by the respiration rate.	V_E can be normal in emphysema; decreased V_E may indicate other diseases, such as pulmonary edema.
Inspiratory reserve volume (IRV) (amount of air inspired above normal inspiration)	Subtract V_T from inspiratory capacity (IC).	Abnormal IRV alone doesn't indicate respiratory dysfunction; IRV decreases during normal exercise.
Expiratory reserve volume (ERV) (amount of air that can be exhaled after normal expiration)	Direct spirographic measurement	ERV varies, even in healthy persons.
Residual volume (RV) (amount of air remaining in the lungs after forced expiration)	Subtract ERV from functional residual capacity (FCR).	RV greater than 35% of total lung capacity (TLC) after maximal expiratory effort may indicate obstructive disease, such as emphysema.

Continued

Interpreting Pulmonary Function Tests
Continued

MEASUREMENT OF PULMONARY FUNCTION	METHOD OF CALCULATION	IMPLICATIONS
Vital capacity (VC) (total volume of air that can be exhaled after maximum inspiration)	Direct spirographic measurement, or add V_T, IRV, and ERV	Normal or increased VC with decreased flow rates may indicate any condition that causes a reduction in functional pulmonary tissue, such as pulmonary lesions, pulmonary edema, atelectasis, excision of pulmonary tissue, pulmonary congestion, or obstruction of bronchus. Decreased VC with normal or increased flow rates may indicate decreased respiratory effort resulting from neuromuscular disease, drug overdose, or head injury; decreased thoracic expansion caused by thoracic or upper abdominal incisions, tight dressings, or kyphoscoliosis; or limited movement of diaphragm resulting from gastric distention, pregnancy, ascites, or abdominal tumor.
Inspiratory capacity (IC) (amount of air that can be inhaled after normal expiration)	Direct spirographic measurement, or add IRV and V_T.	Decreased IC indicates restrictive disease.

Continued

Interpreting Pulmonary Function Tests
Continued

MEASUREMENT OF PULMONARY FUNCTION	METHOD OF CALCULATION	IMPLICATIONS
Functional residual capacity (FRC) (Amount of air remaining in lungs after normal expiration)	Helium dilution technique measurement, or add ERV and RV	Increased FRC indicates overdistention of lungs, which may result from obstructive pulmonary disease.
Total lung capacity (TLC) (total volume of the lungs when maximally inflated)	Add V_T, IRV, ERV, and RV; or FRC and IC; or VC and RV.	Low TLC indicates restrictive disease; high TLC indicates overdistended lungs associated with obstructive disease.
Forced vital capacity (FVC) (dynamic measurement of the amount of air exhaled after maximum inspiration)	Direct spirographic measurement at 1-, 2-, and 3-second intervals	Decreased FVC indicates flow resistance in respiratory system from obstructive disease.
Forced expiratory volume (FEV) (volume of air expired in the 1st, 2nd, or 3rd second of FVC maneuver)	Direct spirographic measurement; expressed as percentage of FVC	Decreased FEV_1, and increased FEV_2 and FEV_3 may indicate obstructive disease; decreased or normal FEV_1 may indicate restrictive disease.

Continued

Interpreting Pulmonary Function Tests
Continued

MEASUREMENT OF PULMONARY FUNCTIONS	METHOD OF CALCULATION	IMPLICATIONS
Maximal mid-expiratory flow (MMEF) **[Also called forced expiratory flow (FEF)]** (average rate of flow during middle half of FVC)	Calculated from the flow rate and the time needed for expiration of middle 50% of FVC	Low MMEF indicates obstructive pulmonary disease.
Maximal voluntary ventilation (MVV) **[Also called maximum breathing capacity (MBC)]** (greatest volume of air breathed per unit of time)	Direct spirographic measurement	Decreased MVV may indicate obstructive disease or restrictive disease, such as myasthenia gravis.
Diffusing capacity for carbon monoxide (DL$_{CO}$) (milliliters of carbon monoxide diffused per minute across the alveolar-capillary membrane)	Calculated from analysis of amount of carbon monoxide exhaled compared with amount inhaled	Decreased DL$_{CO}$ in the presence of thickened alveolar-capillary membrane indicates interstitial pulmonary disease, such as pulmonary fibrosis.

ASSESSING THE PATIENT

Measuring Peak Flow Rate

Peak flow rate—the highest flow point during maximal expiration—helps determine the extent of obstructive disease or bronchospasm. Measurement of peak flow rate, however, may precipitate or worsen bronchospasm. This measurement can also be made before and after bronchodilator administration or respiratory therapy *to gauge the effectiveness of treatment.* The patient can also be instructed how to perform this procedure at home, to monitor airway obstruction. A fall in the peak flow rate may indicate that the patient's condition is deteriorating.

To measure peak flow rate, first obtain a flowmeter, disposable mouthpiece, and a predicted values table. Then, wash your hands. Next, attach a clean mouthpiece to the flowmeter, and press the release button behind the mouthpiece to set the pointer on the flowmeter at zero.

● Explain the procedure to the patient *to ensure his cooperation,* (essential to accurate results).
● Have the patient sit upright in a bed or chair. Then, ask him to inhale as deeply as possible. Tell him to insert the mouthpiece and to seal his lips tightly around it.
● Instruct him to exhale forcefully in one short, sharp blast. Complete emptying of the lungs isn't necessary, *because peak flow is achieved within the first half second of expiration.*
● Remove the mouthpiece, and tell the patient to relax. Then, note the reading on the dial (each mark equals 5 liters). Record peak flow as the observed number or the percentage of predicted peak flow.
● Repeat the test twice, after resetting the pointer.
● Record any adverse effects during the test, such as wheezing or coughing.

Nursing Tip

Instruct the patient scheduled for pulmonary function tests not to eat a heavy meal before the tests and not to smoke for 4 to 6 hours before the tests. Explain the nature and operation of a spirometer. Assure the patient that the procedure is painless and that he can rest between tests.

Don't sedate the patient before the tests. Inform the pulmonary function laboratory if the patient is taking an analgesic that depresses respiration. As ordered, withhold bronchodilator medication for 4 to 6 hours before the tests. Check with the doctor and therapist concerning withholding intermittent positive-pressure breathing therapy.

Some Clinical Implications of Chest X-Rays

NORMAL ANATOMIC LOCATION AND APPEARANCE	POSSIBLE ABNORMALITY	POSSIBLE IMPLICATIONS
Trachea Visible midline in the anterior mediastinal cavity; translucent tubelike appearance	• Deviation from midline • Narrowing, with hourglass appearance and deviation to one side	• Tension pneumo-thorax, atelectasis, pleural effusion, consolidation, mediastinal nodes, or in children, enlarged thymus • Substernal thyroid
Heart Visible in the anterior, left mediastinal cavity; solid appearance due to blood contents; edges may be clear in contrast with surrounding air density of the lung	• Shift • Hypertrophy of right heart • Cardiac borders obscured by stringy densities ("shaggy heart")	• Atelectasis • Cor pulmonale, congestive heart failure • Cystic fibrosis
Aortic knob Visible as water density; formed by the arch of the aorta	• Metal densities (possible calcifications with aorta) • Tortuous shape	• Atherosclerosis • Atherosclerosis
Spine Visible midline in the posterior chest; straight bony structure	• Spinal curvature • Break or misalignment	• Scoliosis, kyphosis • Fractures

Continued

Some Clinical Implications of Chest X-Rays
Continued

NORMAL ANATOMIC LOCATION AND APPEARANCE	POSSIBLE ABNORMALITY	POSSIBLE IMPLICATIONS
Mediastinum (mediastinal shadow) Visible as the space between the lungs; shadowy appearance that widens at the hilum of the lungs	• Deviation to the nondiseased side; deviation toward the diseased side by traction • Gross widening	• Pleural effusion or tumor, fibrosis or collapsed lung • Neoplasms of esophagus, bronchi, lungs, thyroid, lymphoid tissue; aortic aneurysm; mediastinitis; cor pulmonale
Ribs Visible as thoracic cavity encasement	• Break or misalignment • Widening of intercostal spaces	• Fractured sternum or ribs • Emphysema
Clavicles Visible in upper thorax; intact and equidistant in X-ray	• Break or misalignment	• Fractures
Hila (lung roots) Visible above heart where pulmonary vessels, bronchi, and lymph nodes join lungs; appear as small, white, bilateral densities	• Shift to one side • Accentuated shadows	• Atelectasis • Emphysema, pulmonary abscess, tumor, enlarged lymph nodes

Continued

Some Clinical Implications of Chest X-Rays
Continued

NORMAL ANATOMIC LOCATION AND APPEARANCE	POSSIBLE ABNORMALITY	POSSIBLE IMPLICATIONS
Mainstem bronchus Visible to about 1″ (2.5 cm) from hila; translucent, tubelike appearance	• Spherical or oval density	• Bronchogenic cyst
Bronchi Usually not visible	• Visible	• Bronchial pneumonia
Lung fields Usually not visible throughout, except for fine white areas from the hilum	• Visible • Irregular, patchy densities	• Atelectasis • Resolving pneumonia, silicosis, fibrosis, metastatic neoplasm
Hemidiaphragm Rounded, visible; right side ⅜″ to ¾″ (1 to 2 cm) higher than left	• Elevation of diaphragm (difference in elevation can be measured on inspiration and expiration to detect movement) • Flattening of diaphragm • Unilateral elevation of either side	• Active tuberculosis, pneumonia, pleurisy, acute bronchitis, active disease of the abdominal viscera, bilateral phrenic nerve involvement, atelectasis • Asthma, emphysema • Possible pneumothorax or unilateral pulmonary infection, unilateral phrenic nerve paresis

X-Rays and Tissue Density

In a chest X-ray, a high-voltage current passing through a Coolidge tube produces short-wavelength "X" rays. These rays either pass through the chest and react on a photographic plate as light does on film or are partially or fully absorbed by body structures of varying densities before reaching the plate.

Those internal structures filled with gas, like the lungs and airways, allow nearly all X-rays to pass through them and burn into the photographic plate, creating the darkest areas on the film. Tissue with the density of water absorbs some X-rays and prevents them from reaching the film, creating deep gray areas. Bony structures absorb nearly all the X-rays, leaving white or underexposed areas on the film.

Abnormalities appear as changes in normal densities. Since normal pulmonary tissue is radiolucent, foreign bodies, infiltrates, fluids, tumors, and other abnormalities show as white spots in a normally dark area.

Limitations of Chest X-Rays

Although chest X-ray was once routinely performed as a cancer-screening test, the associated risk of exposure to radiation has caused many authorities to question its usefulness. The American Cancer Society now recommends sputum analysis over X-ray.

An X-ray may appear normal in patients with bronchial asthma or chronic bronchitis, even in its severe form, and in patients with emphysema until they reach an advanced stage. Chest X-rays appear normal when respiratory insufficiency stems from extrapulmonary abnormalities, such as brain and spinal cord damage, unless pulmonary infection is present; from neuromuscular disorders (poliomyelitis, myasthenia gravis); and from respiratory depression resulting from sedative overdose. In addition, chest X-rays usually fail to detect primary lung cancer until the tumor has grown to 1 cm in diameter, a process that may take 10 years, and may even overlook large tumors if they're growing in "blind" areas of lung tissue hidden by the heart, great vessels, diaphragm, or other solid organ. Because accurate diagnosis depends on correlating X-ray findings with other radiologic and pulmonary tests, such tests as tomography and ultrasonography may compensate for X-ray's shortcomings.

Common Radiographic Views

Frontal
Performed with the X-ray beam positioned posteriorly and anteriorly and with the patient in an upright position. Posteroanterior (PA) view is the most common frontal view, and is preferred over anteroposterior (AP) view because the heart is anteriorly situated in the thorax and magnified less in a PA view than in an AP view. The frontal views show greater lung area than the other views because of the lower diaphragm position.

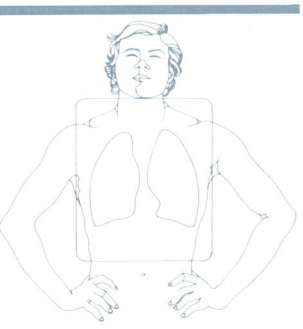

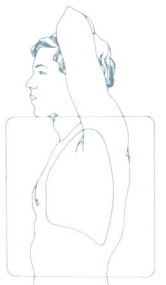

Lateral
Performed with the X-ray beam directed toward the patient's side. the left lateral (LL) view is the most common lateral view, and is preferred over the right lateral (RL) view because the heart is left of midline and magnified less in a LL view than in a RL view. Lateral views visualize lesions not apparent on a PA view.

Recumbent
Performed with the X-ray beam overhead and with the patient in a supine position. This view helps distinguish free fluid from encapsulated fluid and from an elevated diaphragm.

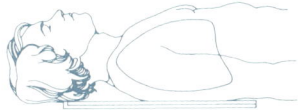

Continued

Common Radiographic Views
Continued

Oblique

Performed with the X-ray beam angled between the frontal and lateral views. This view helps evaluate intrathoracic disorders (such as pleural effusion), esophageal abnormalities, and mediastinal masses. (Rarely, it is also used to localize lesions within the chest.)

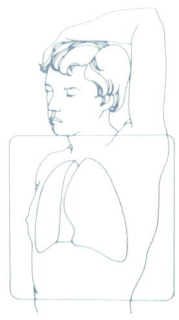

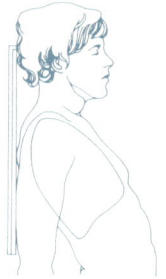

Lordotic

Performed with the X-ray beam directed through the axis of the middle thoracic lobe and with the patient leaning back against the film plate. This view evaluates the collapse of the area or the presence of pleural fluid.

Decubitus

Performed with the X-ray beam parallel to the floor and with the patient in one of several horizontal positions (supine, prone, or side). This view demonstrates the extent of pulmonary abscess or cavity, the presence of free pleural fluid or pneumothorax, and the mobility of mediastinal mass when the patient changes positions.

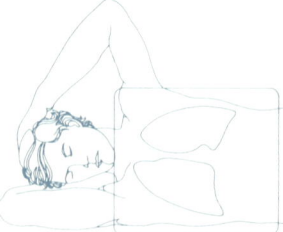

Positioning the Patient for Thoracentesis

To prepare the patient for thoracentesis, place him in one of the three positions shown below: (1) sitting on the edge of the bed with arms on overbed table; (2) sitting up in bed with arms on overbed table; (3) lying partially on the side, partially on the back with arms over the head. These positions serve to widen the intercostal spaces and permit easy access to the pleural cavity. Using pillows as shown will make the patient more comfortable.

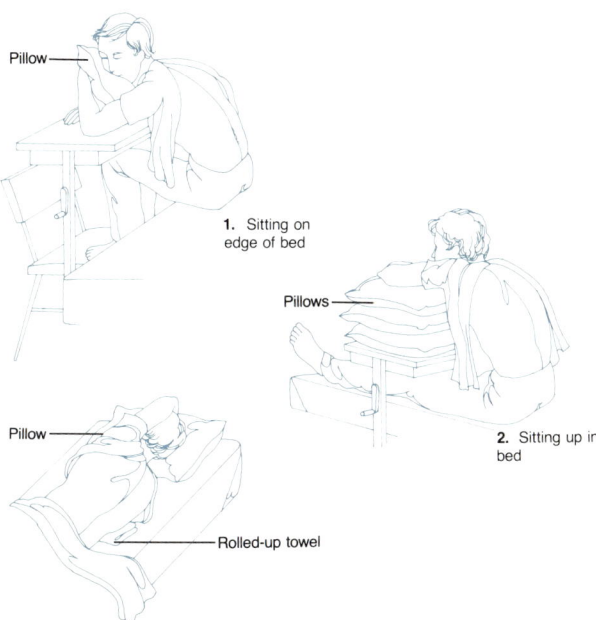

Pillow

1. Sitting on edge of bed

Pillows

2. Sitting up in bed

Pillow

Rolled-up towel

3. Lying partially on side, partially on back

After Thoracentesis: How to Care for the Patient

Caring for your patient. After the procedure's over, watch your patient closely for possible complications. Check for lung tissue damage by observing his sputum for traces of blood. Watch for pneumothorax by checking his vital signs and breath sounds at least once every 30 minutes.

Signs and symptoms of pneumothorax include increased respiratory rate, increased pulse rate, blood pressure changes, skin color changes, asymmetric chest expansion, dyspnea, chest pain, and diminished or absent breath sounds on the affected side. If you strongly suspect a pneumothorax, notify the doctor immediately and begin giving the patient oxygen. The doctor will probably order a portable chest X-ray exam. If the results confirm a pneumothorax, be prepared to help insert chest tubes.

Charting. Document the procedure, including the doctor's name, time when the procedure began and ended, and color and amount of pleural fluid obtained. Indicate whether you sent specimens to the lab, as well as which studies the doctor ordered. Also indicate how well your patient tolerated the procedure; record his vital signs both before and after thoracentesis. Finally, be sure to include date, time, and your signature.

Caring for laboratory specimens. Send specimen containers to the lab promptly. Make sure they're correctly labeled with your patient's name, room number, and doctor's name. Remember, some tests require warm specimens; others may require biopsy specimens in saline solution or formalin. To make sure specimens are usable when they get to the lab, check first with laboratory personnel for instructions.

Caring for equipment. Dispose of needles and syringes correctly. Discard all nonreusable materials. Did the doctor use a biopsy needle? Carefully clean it and return it intact to central supply for sterilization and recycling.

Recognizing Complications of Thoracentesis

Identify the following possible complications of thoracentesis by watching for their characteristic signs and symptoms:

• *pneumothorax:* apprehension, increased restlessness, cyanosis, tachycardia, absent or diminished breath sounds on the affected side

• *tension pneumothorax:* dyspnea, chest pain, tachycardia, deviated trachea

• *fluid reaccumulation:* increasing and persistent cough, respiratory distress, hemoptysis, subcutaneous emphysema

• *mediastinal shift:* labored breathing, cardiac dysrhythmias, cardiac distress, pulmonary edema (pink, frothy sputum, paradoxical pulse).

Interpreting Results of Thoracentesis

Pleural effusion results from the abnormal formation or reabsorption of pleural fluid. Certain characteristics classify pleural fluid as either a transudate (a low-protein fluid that has leaked from normal blood vessels) or an exudate (a protein-rich fluid that has leaked from blood vessels with increased permeability).

Transudative effusion generally results from diminished colloidal pressure, increased negative pressure within the pleural cavity, ascites, systemic and pulmonary venous hypertension, congestive heart failure, hepatic cirrhosis, and nephritis.

Exudative effusion results from disorders that increase pleural capillary permeability (possibly with changes in hydrostatic or colloid osmotic pressures), lymphatic drainage interference, infections, pulmonary infarctions, and neoplasms. Exudative effusion associated with depressed glucose levels, elevated LDH, rheumatoid arthritis cells, and negative smears, cultures, and cytologic examination may indicate pleurisy associated with rheumatoid arthritis.

Examining Pleural Fluid

CHARACTERISTIC	POSSIBLE CAUSE
Light, straw-colored	• Normal
Purulent	• Empyema
Blood-tinged	• Hemothorax • Tuberculosis • Pulmonary infarction • Neoplastic disease • Accidental tissue damage from thoracentesis
Milky	• Chylothorax • Invasion of thoracic duct by a tumor, or an inflammatory process • Traumatic rupture of thoracic duct • Cellular debris or cholesterol crystals
Low-protein fluid (transudate)	• Cirrhosis • Congestive heart disease
Protein-rich fluid (exudate)	• Infectious disease • Asbestosis • Pulmonary infarction • Lymphatic drainage disorder

Nursing Tip

On the patient's chart, document the color and amount of pleural fluid obtained, and indicate which studies the doctor ordered. Also note how well the patient tolerated the procedure.

Significance of Pleural Fluid Analysis

GRAM STAIN CULTURE AND SENSITIVITY

Interpretation

Positive result may mean the early stages of bacterial infection. In the later stages of bacterial infection, the fluid may look grossly purulent with a positive Gram stain, yet cultures may be negative from antibiotic therapy.

ACID-FAST STAIN AND CULTURE

Interpretation

Positive result may indicate tuberculosis.

RED BLOOD CELL COUNT

Interpretation

If count is about 10,000/mm^3 and the specimen's pink or light red, may indicate tissue damage. If count is above 100,000/mm^3 and the specimen's grossly bloody, suggests intrapleural malignancy, pulmonary infarction, tuberculosis, or closed chest trauma. If a hemothorax is present, the hematocrit of the pleural fluid will be similar to that of capillary blood.

LEUKOCYTE COUNT

Interpretation

If count is above 1,000/mm^3 or above 50% neutrophils, may indicate septic or nonseptic inflammation.

LYMPHOCYTE COUNT

Interpretation

If count is over 50%, may indicate tuberculosis, lymphoma, or other form of cancer.

BLOOD CLOTS

Interpretation

May indicate neoplasm, tuberculosis, or infection.

Continued

Significance of Pleural Fluid Analysis
Continued

SPECIFIC GRAVITY

Interpretation
If measurement exceeds 1.016, may indicate neoplasm, tuberculosis, or infection; if less than 1.104, may indicate congestive heart failure.

TOTAL PROTEIN

Interpretation
Level below 3 g/dl may indicate congestive heart failure or other transudates. Level above 3 g/dl suggests neoplasm, tuberculosis, or infection.

LACTIC DEHYDROGENASE (LDH)

Interpretation
Levels rise in cancer and other conditions associated with exudates; decrease in heart failure and other conditions associated with transudates.

GLUCOSE

Interpretation
If less than serum glucose level, may suggest cancer, bacterial infection, or nonseptic inflammation.

SEDIMENT

Interpretation
May represent cancerous cells, cellular debris, or cholesterol crystals.

BIOPSY

Interpretation
May reveal a tumor.

Special Consideration

To prevent hypovolemic shock, fluid is removed slowly and no more than 1,200 ml of fluid is removed at one time.

Pleuritic or shoulder pain may indicate pleural irritation by the needle point.

A chest X-ray is usually ordered after the procedure to detect pneumothorax and evaluate the results of the procedure.

Performing Bronchoscopy

The bronchoscopic tube, inserted through the nostril into the bronchi, has four channels (see inset). Two light channels (A) provide a light source: one visualizing channel (B) to see through and one open channel (C) that accommodates biopsy forceps, cytology brush, suctioning, lavage, anesthetic, or oxygen.

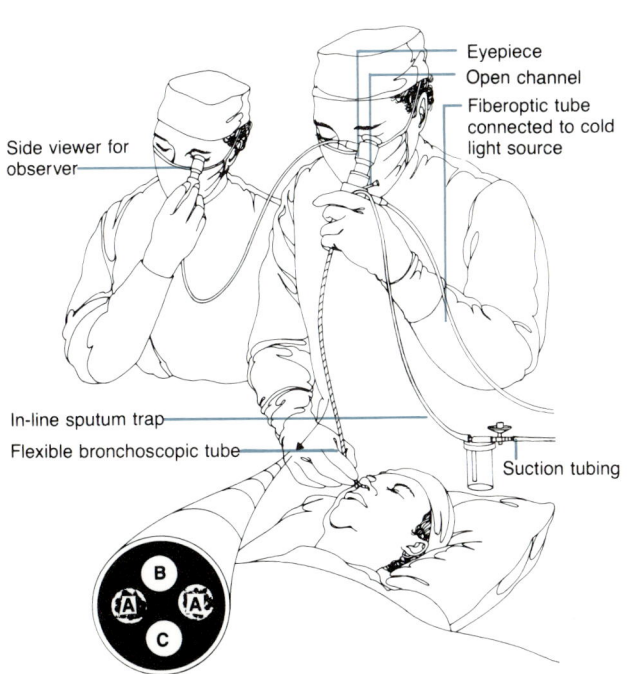

Side viewer for observer

Eyepiece
Open channel
Fiberoptic tube connected to cold light source

In-line sputum trap
Flexible bronchoscopic tube

Suction tubing

Patient Care after Bronchoscopy

After bronchoscopy, monitor vital signs every 15 minutes or as ordered, until they are stable. Notify the doctor immediately of any complications or deterioration in the patient's condition. Keep resuscitative equipment and tracheotomy tray available for 24 hours after the test.

As ordered, place the conscious patient in the semi-Fowler's position; place the unconscious patient on his side, with the head of the bed slightly elevated to prevent aspiration. Provide an emesis basin, and instruct the patient to spit out saliva rather than swallow it. Sputum may be blood-tinged. Notify the doctor if excessive bleeding occurs. Collect sputum for 24 hours immediately following a bronchoscopy for cytologic studies and culture.

Instruct the patient to refrain from clearing his throat and coughing, which may dislodge the clot at a biopsy site and cause hemorrhage. Also, advise the patient to avoid smoking for the rest of the day of the procedure, because it irritates the tissues.

Restrict food and fluids until after the gag reflex returns (usually in 1½ to 2 hours, although it may take longer in some patients). To test for return of gag reflex, touch the back of his throat with a tongue blade. Also, if the patient has had general anesthesia, check for bowel sounds. Only after bowel sounds and gag reflex have returned should the patient begin to take oral nourishment, as ordered. Usually, you can offer ice chips, then water, and within a few hours, his usual diet. Also, provide medicated lozenges, as ordered, or a local anesthetic to ease discomfort. To prevent laryngeal edema, provide humidification, as ordered.

Reassure the patient that hoarseness and sore throat are only temporary, and encourage him to avoid straining his voice.

Collecting a Sputum Culture

Use these guidelines to help you collect a sputum specimen that can be accurately analyzed by the laboratory:

• Collect the specimen first thing in the morning, if possible. Have the patient brush his teeth and rinse his mouth before coughing into sputum cup.

• Make sure the patient coughs deeply enough. If you're using a suction catheter, make sure it extends all the way to the bronchus.

• Collect at least 5 cc.

• If the patient has a contagious disease, collect the sputum specimen in a nonporous container and label it "contaminated."

• Take the specimen to the lab immediately.

Analyzing a Sputum Specimen

Four types of tests may be performed on a sputum specimen to identify the infecting organism or abnormal cells.

Gram stain differentiates gram-positive bacteria, which retain the crystal or Gentian violet stain after decolorization, from gram-negative bacteria, which lose the violet stain but counterstain red with safranine. The test permits rapid visualization of bacteria from a smear and indicates if the specimen is representative (many white blood cells, few epithelial cells) or if oral contamination has occurred (few WBCs, many epithelial cells). Gram staining often provides early presumptive diagnosis of lower respiratory infection, such as bacterial pneumonia.

Acid-fast stain helps rapidly identify organisms of the genus *Mycobacterium,* since they retain carbolfuchsin stain after treatment with an acid-alcohol solution. This test provides early presumptive diagnosis of tuberculosis.

Culture and sensitivity testing allows growth and isolation of microbes for positive identification and determination of their vulnerability to specific antibiotics. The test helps diagnose lower respiratory infection or confirm earlier presumptive diagnosis from a stained smear.

Cytologic (exfoliative) testing is performed to identify cancer cells and other abnormal cells to help diagnose and type malignant pulmonary lesions and identify granulomas, inflammation, and other benign conditions.

Checking for Cardiac Involvement

If your patient's in respiratory distress, the doctor may order an EKG to check for cardiac problems caused or exacerbated by the respiratory crisis. For example, if your patient has a preexisting dysrhythmia that increases his body's oxygen demand, an acute respiratory disorder could cause a *cardiac* crisis.

An EKG can also provide important clues about the respiratory disorder. For instance, sinus tachycardia, a relatively minor dysrhythmia, may be the first sign of pulmonary embolism.

Cardiac dysrhythmias that may accompany a respiratory emergency include:
• supraventricular tachycardia
• atrial fibrillation
• ventricular irritability (possibly progressing to ventricular tachycardia).

The chart below shows which respiratory disorders may cause a specific dysrhythmia and describes each dysrhythmia's EKG features.

SINUS TACHYCARDIA

Respiratory cause
• Possibly the first sign of pulmonary embolism
EKG features and significance
• Rate is 100 to 160 beats/minute. (Tracing shows 130 beats/minute.)
• Impulse formation and conduction are normal.
• Prolonged sinus tachycardia may lead to ischemia and myocardial damage by raising oxygen requirements.

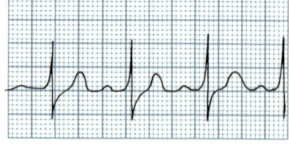

PREMATURE ATRIAL CONTRACTION (PAC)

Respiratory cause
• Acute respiratory failure or COPD
EKG features and significance
• Premature, occasionally abnormal P waves
• QRS complexes follow, except in very early or blocked PACs.
• P wave may be buried in the preceding T wave.
• Premature beat may be conducted aberrantly, as shown.

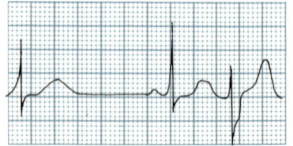

Continued

Checking for Cardiac Involvement
Continued

PAROXYSMAL SUPRAVENTRIC-
ULAR TACHYCARDIA (PSVT)
OR PAROXYSMAL ATRIAL
TACHYCARDIA

Respiratory cause
• Hypoxemia
EKG features and significance
• Heart rate > 140 beats/minute;
rarely exceeds 250 beats/minute
• P waves are regular but aber-
rant; difficult to differentiate from
preceding T wave.
• PSVT may cause palpitations,
light-headedness, and exhaustion.

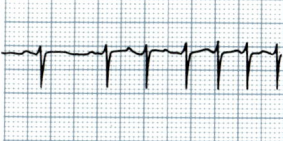

ATRIAL FLUTTER

Respiratory cause
• Pulmonary embolism
EKG features and significance
• Ventricular rate (usually 60 to
100 beats/minute) depends on
degree of AV block and is usually
regular.
• Atrial rate is 250 to 400 beats/
minute and usually regular.
• QRS complexes are uniform in
shape; may be regular or irregular, depending on the degree of
AV block.

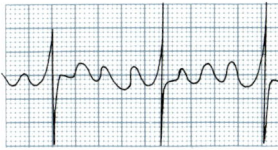

Continued

Checking for Cardiac Involvement
Continued

PREMATURE VENTRICULAR
CONTRACTION (PVC)

Respiratory cause
● Hypoxemia, as in respiratory
failure
EKG features and significance
● Focus can be unifocal (same
appearance in every lead) or mul-
tifocal.
● Beat occurs prematurely, usually followed by a complete compensatory pause.
● QRS complex is wide (> 0.14
second) and distorted.
● Dysrhythmia can occur singly,
in pairs, or in threes.

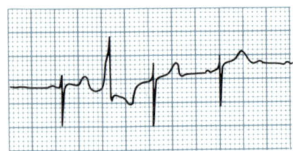

THIRD-DEGREE AV BLOCK
(COMPLETE HEART BLOCK)

Respiratory cause
● Hypoxemia
EKG features and significance
● Atrial impulses are blocked at
AV node; atrial and ventricular im-
pulses dissociated; no relationship
between P waves and QRS com-
plexes
● Atrial rate is regular; ventricular
rate is slow and regular.
● Irregular PR interval
● QRS complex may be normal or
wide.

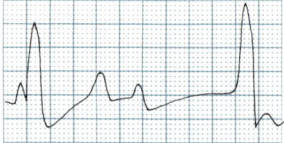

Determining the Chief Complaint

Record the patient's description of his chief complaint. The most common chief complaints in patients with respiratory disorders are cough—with or without sputum production or hemoptysis—dyspnea, and chest pain.

When you have identified the patient's chief complaint, define his illness in greater detail by asking the following types of questions:

Cough. *Does your cough usually occur at a specific time of day? How does it sound—dry, hacking, barking, congested?* Try to determine whether the patient's cough is related to cigarette smoking or other irritants. (Usually coughing results from smoking or chronic bronchitis.)

Are you taking any drug or receiving treatment to clear the cough? If so, how often? Have you recently been exposed to anyone with a similar cough? Was that person's cough caused by a cold or flu?

Sputum production. *How much sputum are you coughing up per day?* Remember, the tracheobronchial tree can produce up to 3 oz (90 ml) of sputum per day.

What time of day do you cough up the most sputum? Smokers cough the most in the morning; nonsmokers generally don't. Coughing from an irritant occurs most often during exposure to it.

Is sputum production increasing? This may result from external stimuli or from such internal causes as chronic bronchial infection. Excess production of sputum that separates into layers may indicate bronchiectasis.

Does the sputum contain mucus or look frothy? What color is it? Has its color changed? Does it smell bad? Foul-smelling sputum may result from an anaerobic infection, such as an abscess. Blood-tinged or rust-colored sputum may result from trauma caused by coughing or from such underlying conditions as bronchitis, pulmonary infarction or infections, tuberculosis, and tumors. A color change from white to yellow or green indicates infection.

Dyspnea. *Are you always short of breath, or do you have*
Continued

CONTROLLING RESPIRATORY DISORDERS

Determining the Chief Complaint
Continued

intermittent attacks of breath-lessness? Onset of dyspnea may be slow or abrupt.

What relieves the attacks— repositioning yourself, relaxing, taking medication? Do the attacks cause your lips and nail beds to turn blue? Does body position, time of day, or any activity affect your breathing? Paroxysmal nocturnal dyspnea and orthopnea are commonly associated with cardiac dysfunction but may be related to chronic lung disease.

How many stairs can you climb, or how many blocks can you walk, before you begin to feel short of breath? Do such activities as taking a shower or shopping make you feel that way? Dyspnea that follows activity suggests poor ventilation or perfusion, or inefficient breathing mechanisms.

Do you experience any associated discomfort, such as cough, unusual sweating, or chest pain? Does the breathlessness seem to be stable or getting worse? Is it accompanied by external sounds, *such as wheezing or stridor?* Wheezing results from small-airway obstruction (for example, from an aspirated foreign body). Stridor results from tracheal compression or laryngeal edema.

Chest pain. *Is the pain localized? Is it constant, or do you experience attacks? Have you ever had a chest injury? Does a specific activity (such as movement of the upper body or exercise) produce pain?* Respiratory disorders usually cause musculoskeletal chest pain; that is, pain related to motion. (Remember, the lungs have no pain-sensitive nerves; however, the parietal pleura and the tracheobronchial tree do.) Of course, chest pain is also commonly associated with cardiovascular disorders.

Is the pain accompanied by other discomfort such as coughing, sneezing, or shortness of breath? Does splinting relieve the pain? Does the pain occur when you breathe normally, or only when you breathe deeply? Pain on deep breathing is often pleuritic.

Classifying Respiratory Signs and Symptoms

CLASSIFICATION/ DYSPNEA	COUGHING	SPUTUM PRODUCTION
None/During strenuous exercise	Occasionally with colds	Only with colds
Slight or mild/ While hurrying on a level surface or walking up a slight incline (able to walk at a normal pace on level ground)	Occasionally in morning	Occasionally in morning
Moderate/While walking for some time on a level surface (able to walk about 1 mile at his own pace)	Four to six times daily	Twice daily, 4 or more days a week
Severe to very severe/After walking about 100 yards or a few minutes on a level surface. Very severe/ Breathlessness during routine activities; confined to the house because of dyspnea	Throughout the day for at least 3 consecutive months	Throughout the day for at least 3 consecutive months

Guide to Respiratory Disorders

CHEST WALL DEFORMITIES (INCLUDING PECTUS EXCAVATUM, KYPHOSCOLIOSIS, THORACOPLASTY, AND TRAUMA)

Chief complaint
- *Cough:* absent or productive, depending on severity or tendency toward infection
- *Dyspnea:* present only in severe deformity
- *Chest pain:* absent

History
- Possibly asymptomatic; signs and symptoms occur gradually; past history of chest trauma or congenital deformity

Physical examination and diagnostic studies
- Physical deformities; accessory muscle changes; lung distortion, making interpretation of findings difficult; flail chest (paradoxical movement of region of wall and local bulging during expiration, and retraction during inspiration); consolidation may be present; no adventitious sounds
- Chest X-ray and pulmonary function test normal or abnormal, depending on severity of deformity; chronic deformity may cause increase in hematocrit and hemoglobin (polycythemia)

OBESITY, PICKWICKIAN SYNDROME

Chief complaint
- *Cough:* absent or productive, depending on severity or tendency toward infection
- *Dyspnea:* absent, or present only on exertion
- *Chest pain:* absent

History
- Possibly asymptomatic; history of weight gain; daytime somnolence

Physical examination and diagnostic studies
- Distant breath sounds; reduced respiratory excursion
- Possible abnormal pulmonary function test

PNEUMONECTOMY

Chief complaint
- *Cough:* absent
- *Dyspnea:* absent, unless remaining portion of lung is unable to compensate
- *Chest pain:* absent

History
- Possibly asymptomatic; history of lung surgery; fatigue

Physical examination and diagnostic studies
- Breath sounds absent; in partial pneumonectomy, remaining portion of lung may overexpand,

Continued

Guide to Respiratory Disorders
Continued

PNEUMONECTOMY
Continued

causing hyperresonance; in total pneumonectomy, decreased respiratory excursion occurs on affected side
● Chest X-ray and pulmonary function test normal or abnormal, depending on severity of deformity

TUMOR

Chief complaint
● *Cough:* present; cardinal symptom of bronchial tumor or of tumor compressing bronchus
● *Dyspnea:* usually present if tumor is large
● *Chest pain:* possibly pleuritic or dull
History
● Presence of signs and symptoms depends on tumor's size and location
Physical examination and diagnostic studies
● In large tumor, physical findings same as those of chronic pleural effusion
● Chest X-ray abnormal

PLEURAL EFFUSION (SMALL, ACUTE)

Chief complaint
● *Cough:* absent
● *Dyspnea:* possible

● *Chest pain:* possibly pleuritic or dull
History
● Possibly asymptomatic; history of neoplasms, congestive heart failure, rheumatoid arthritis, subphrenic abscess, pancreatitis
Physical examination and diagnostic studies
● Limited respiratory excursion may be present; tactile fremitus decreased or absent; dull percussion; decreased breath and voice sounds; adventitious sounds caused by underlying pathology
● Chest X-ray abnormal

PLEURAL EFFUSION (LARGE, CHRONIC)

Chief complaint
● *Cough:* absent
● *Dyspnea:* usually present
● *Chest pain:* possibly pleuritic or dull
History
● Possibly symptomatic; same history as small, acute pleural effusion
Physical examination and diagnostic studies
● Trachea deviates toward normal side; tactile fremitus absent; dull or flat percussion; voice sounds absent or decreased; breath sounds absent; adventitious sounds caused by underlying pathology and lung consolidation
● Chest X-ray abnormal

Continued

Guide to Respiratory Disorders
Continued

NEUROMUSCULAR DISORDERS

Chief complaint
• *Cough:* absent
• *Dyspnea:* possible
• *Chest pain:* absent
History
• *Neuromuscular disorders:* medulla or spinal cord dysfunction, bulbar poliomyelitis, cervical cord trauma, Guillain-Barré syndrome, muscular dystrophy, myasthenia gravis
• *Respiratory center depression:* brain tumor, sedation, industrial or carbon monoxide poisoning, polymyxin or other antibiotic therapy, encephalopathy, high-flow uncontrolled oxygen therapy
Physical examination and diagnostic studies
• Shallow or absent respiration, requiring artificial ventilation; distant breath sounds; respiratory muscle atrophy; adventitious sounds caused by underlying pathology; symptoms of neuromuscular disease
• Pulmonary function test abnormal; arterial blood gas analysis may be abnormal

CLOSED PNEUMOTHORAX

Chief complaint
• *Cough:* absent
• *Dyspnea:* moderate

• *Chest pain:* pleuritic; may be sudden and sharp
History
• Dizziness, emphysema, tuberculosis
Physical examination and diagnostic studies
• Crepitus; if small, no trachea deviation; *on affected side:* limited respiratory excursion; tactile fremitus absent; resonant or hyperresonant percussion; breath and voice sounds absent or decreased; no adventitious sounds
• Chest X-ray abnormal

OPEN PNEUMOTHORAX

Chief complaint
• *Cough:* absent
• *Dyspnea:* severe
• *Chest pain:* severe, pleuritic; sudden and sharp
History
• Dizziness
Physical examination and diagnostic studies
• Crepitus; trachea deviates to normal side; *on affected side:* limited respiratory excursion; tactile fremitus absent; hyperresonant or tympanic percussion; breath and voice sounds absent or decreased; no adventitious sounds; cyanosis
• Chest X-ray abnormal

Continued

Guide to Respiratory Disorders
Continued

TENSION PNEUMOTHORAX

Chief complaint
- *Cough:* absent
- *Dyspnea:* severe
- *Chest pain:* severe, pleuritic; sudden and sharp

History
- Acute symptoms

Physical examination and diagnostic studies
- Cyanosis; shock; possible tympanic percussion; other physical findings same as those of open pneumothorax
- Chest X-ray abnormal

ASTHMATIC ATTACK

Chief complaint
- *Cough:* dry and minimal; progresses to thick and productive
- *Dyspnea:* severe, with audible wheezing
- *Chest pain:* absent

History
- *Allergic asthma:* history of taking aspirin or other nonsteroidal anti-inflammatory agents; exposure to feathers, dander, molds, or certain foods; family history of allergies
- *Idiosyncratic asthma:* attacks common following respiratory infection; no family history of allergies
- *Precipitating or exacerbating asthma:* environment, stress, occupation, exercise, respiratory infection

Physical examination and diagnostic studies
- Tachycardia; pale and slightly cyanotic appearance; tendency to sit or lean forward; difficult speech; diaphoresis; nasal flaring on expiration; bulging neck veins; use of accessory muscles in retraction of intercostal, supraclavicular, and suprasternal spaces; markedly distended and fixed chest in inspiratory position; tactile fremitus decreased; hyperresonant percussion; diaphragm low on percussion; voice sounds decreased; breath sounds distant; expiration greater than inspiration; sibilant rhonchi (wheezing) throughout lung fields on expiration
- Chest X-ray normal; arterial blood gas analysis abnormal during attack
- Hyperinflation may be present

Continued

Guide to Respiratory Disorders
Continued

CHRONIC OBSTRUCTIVE PULMONARY DISEASE (COPD) TYPE A

Chief complaint
• *Cough:* present, with scant mucoid production
• *Dyspnea:* insidious onset; slowly progresses to severe dyspnea on exertion
• *Chest pain:* absent

History
• Genetic predisposition; cigarette smoking; acute recurring respiratory illness (more common in Type B); exposure to environmental hazards; under age 60

Physical examination and diagnostic studies
• Reddish complexion; weight loss; neck veins distended on expiration, collapsed on inspiration; increased anteroposterior diameter; use of accessory muscles; decreased respiratory excursion bilaterally; decreased tactile fremitus; hyperresonant percussion; decreased diaphragmatic excursion; breath sounds distant with prolonged expiration; pursed lips when breathing; decreased voice sounds; adventitious sounds; occasionally wheezing
• Chest X-ray abnormal; pulmonary function test abnormal; arterial blood gas analysis abnormal; hematocrit abnormal

CHRONIC OBSTRUCTIVE PULMONARY DISEASE (COPD) TYPE B

Chief complaint
• *Cough:* chronic and productive cough occurring most often in the morning, for at least 3 months of the year for 2 consecutive years; possibly hemoptysis
• *Dyspnea:* first occurs only during chest infections; less severe than Type A
• *Chest pain:* absent, except in second-degree chronic cough

History
• Exposure to air pollution, inorganic and/or organic dusts, or noxious gases; cigarette smoking; genetic predisposition; increased frequency of respiratory infections

Physical examination and diagnostic studies
• Cyanosis; overweight; increased anteroposterior chest diameter (barrel chest); hyperresonance on percussion; prolonged expiratory phase; sibilant and sonorous rhonchi and rales (crackles) may be present; cor pulmonale may occur as complication
• Chest X-ray normal or abnormal (may show evidence of past inflammatory disease); pulmonary function test abnormal; arterial blood gas analysis abnormal; hematocrit abnormal

Continued

Guide to Respiratory Disorders
Continued

ADVANCED BRONCHIECTASIS

Chief complaint
- *Cough:* chronic, with copious, foul, purulent sputum; hemoptysis
- *Dyspnea:* present in severe and extensive disease
- *Chest pain:* absent, except in pneumonia or second-degree chronic cough

History
- Recurring pneumonia or sinusitis; congenital defects in bronchial system; hereditary predisposition; deficient immunities; local bronchial obstruction; general weakness and fatigue

Physical examination and diagnostic studies
- Cyanosis; clubbing; fever; night sweats; weight loss; sibilant or sonorous rhonchi and crackles over lower lobes; in progressive advanced bronchiectasis, lung findings similar to Type A chronic obstructive pulmonary disease
- Chest X-ray abnormal; bronchography abnormal; pulmonary function test normal or abnormal; arterial blood gas analysis abnormal

MYCOPLASMAL PNEUMONIA (ATYPICAL PNEUMONIA)

Chief complaint
- *Cough:* prolonged history of dry, hacking, possibly persistent cough; no hemoptysis
- *Dyspnea:* absent
- *Chest pain:* present, possibly from secondary musculoskeletal cough

History
- Between age 5 and 20; family history of disease; onset of signs and symptoms resembles that of viral respiratory tract infection (malaise, myalgia, sore throat, headache, mild cough, earache)

Physical examination and diagnostic studies
- Fever during first 2 weeks; in about 15% of cases, inflamed tympanic membrane, with bullae; fine crepitant crackles at end of inspiratory cycle possible; dullness on percussion; rhonchi; coarse or musical wheezes; normal chest findings possible
- Chest X-ray abnormal; complement fixation test shows level of specific antibody to *Mycoplasma;* no leukocytosis

Continued

Guide to Respiratory Disorders
Continued

BACTERIAL PNEUMONIA

Chief complaint
- *Cough:* present, productive, with mucoid, purulent sputum; hemoptysis
- *Dyspnea:* present on exertion
- *Chest pain:* present, pleuritic

History
- Predisposing conditions include depressed cough and glottis reflexes; altered consciousness from alcoholism, drug abuse, seizure, head trauma, general anesthetic, cerebrovascular disease, old age; painful breathing; muscle weakness; neuromuscular diseases; obstructive diseases; impaired mucus transport; possibly aspiration of vomitus or oil; respiration or immunosuppressive drug therapy

Physical examination and diagnostic studies
- Fever, chills, tachycardia, tachypnea, cyanosis, hypotension, guarding and decreased excursion on affected side
- *With adventitious sounds:* crepitant inspiratory crackles, pleural friction rub with pleural involvement
- *With consolidation:* tactile fremitus increased; percussion dull or flat; breath sounds tubular or bronchial; voice sounds increased, including bronchophony, egophony, and whispered pectoriloquy
- *With bronchial plug and consolidation:* tactile fremitus absent; percussion dull; voice, breath sounds decreased or absent
- Increased white blood cell count; chest X-ray abnormal; sputum examination abnormal

LUNG ABSCESS

Chief complaint
- *Cough:* present, productive, with large amounts of bloody, purulent sputum
- *Dyspnea:* present, frequent
- *Chest pain:* present, pleuritic

History
- Recurrent dental infections; history similar to that of bacterial pneumonia but more insidious; history of altered mental status

Physical examination and diagnostic studies
- Fever, weight loss, fetid breath, poor dentition; respiratory findings may appear normal or similar to consolidation in bacterial pneumonia
- Chest X-ray normal or abnormal; sputum culture should identify organism; increased white blood cell count (leukocytosis)

Continued

Guide to Respiratory Disorders
Continued

LUNG TUBERCULOSIS

Chief complaint
- *Cough:* present, productive, purulent; hemoptysis
- *Dyspnea:* present only in advanced disease
- *Chest pain:* present, occasionally pleuritic

History
- Possibly asymptomatic; malaise, irritability at end of day; night sweats; exposure to active pulmonary tuberculosis; associated with uncontrolled diabetes, alcoholism, undernutrition, institutionalization, long-term treatment with corticosteroids

Physical examination and diagnostic studies
- Fever; weight loss; decreased respiratory excursion; in early stages, respiratory findings may appear normal; extensive fibrosis may cause consolidation: apical dullness, bronchial breath sounds, coarse rales
- Chest X-ray abnormal; sputum culture positive for tubercle bacillus; positive tuberculin test

PULMONARY FIBROSIS, NON-CHEMICAL (DUST, INDUSTRIAL IRRITANTS, ALLERGENS)

Chief complaint
- *Cough:* present, dry, irritable, progressing to productive hemoptysis
- *Dyspnea:* present, progressive, exertional; wheezing; tachypnea
- *Chest pain:* present

History
- Inhalation of dust, industrial irritants, or allergens; malaise; weight loss; anorexia

Physical examination and diagnostic studies
- Cyanosis on exertion; fine metallic crepitant basilar rales; decreased chest excursion in advanced disease
- Chest X-ray abnormal; pulmonary function test abnormal

PULMONARY FIBROSIS, CHEMICAL (IRRITANT GASES, CHEMICALS)

Chief complaint
- *Cough:* present, hemoptysis
- *Dyspnea:* present, wheezing
- *Chest pain:* present

History
- Exposure to irritant gases or chemicals

Physical examination and diagnostic studies
- Burning and irritation of eyes, nose, throat, trachea; nausea and vomiting; cyanosis on exertion; fine metallic crepitant basilar rales; decreased chest excursion in advanced disease
- Chest X-ray abnormal; pulmonary function test abnormal

Continued

Guide to Respiratory Disorders
Continued

PULMONARY EDEMA

Chief complaint
• *Cough:* dry at first, progressing to productive, with pink, frothy sputum
• *Dyspnea:* in acute form: wheezing; in chronic form: paroxysmal nocturnal dyspnea; orthopnea
• *Chest pain:* absent
History
• May be sudden or chronic; history of heart disease
Physical examination and diagnostic studies
• *Acute:* must sit up and lean forward to breathe; cyanosis; resonant percussion; normal voice sounds; breath sounds reveal prolonged expiratory phase; adventitious sounds reveal dry, fine crackles usually at base, progressing to moist, bubbling crackles throughout chest; sibilant rhonchi; rattle sound
• *Chronic:* enlarged heart, peripheral edema, hepatomegaly, bilateral diffuse butterfly density from hilum
• Chest X-ray abnormal

CONNECTIVE TISSUE DISEASE AFFECTING THE LUNGS (SUCH AS SYSTEMIC LUPUS ERYTHEMATOSUS)

Chief complaint
• *Cough:* may be present, with or without production
• *Dyspnea:* present
• *Chest pain:* pleuritic or dull sensation, with pleural effusion
History
• Past history of connective tissue disease
Physical examination and diagnostic studies
• Signs of specific suspected disease; fibrosis; clubbing; decreased respiratory excursion; trachea deviates toward more affected side; resonant to dull percussion; decreased breath and voice sounds, especially in diffuse fibrosis; rales audible on inspiration and expiration; pleural friction rub
• Chest X-ray abnormal; pulmonary function tests abnormal; specific tests to identify disease include antinuclear antibody and Rh factor

PULMONARY EMBOLISM

Chief complaint
• *Cough:* hemoptysis
• *Dyspnea:* sudden, unexplained tachypnea
• *Chest pain:* pleuritic, but only if infarction occurs
History
• Previous thromboemboli, recent surgery, dehydration, pregnancy,

Continued

Guide to Respiratory Disorders
Continued

PULMONARY EMBOLISM
Continued

congestive heart failure, chronic pulmonary disease, use of oral contraceptives, leg fracture, deep venous insufficiency, extended inactivity
Physical examination and diagnostic studies
• Tachycardia; may be normal except for rales and localized wheezing; pleural effusion and pleural friction rub possible if infarction occurs; atelectasis and pneumonia may occur as complications
• Chest X-ray inconclusive; ABG's abnormal; pulmonary angiography abnormal. Ventilation/perfusion lung scan abnormal

LUNG TUMOR

Chief complaint
• *Cough:* absent, mild, or change in pattern of chronic cough
• *Dyspnea:* absent or on exertion
• *Chest pain:* absent
History
• May be asymptomatic; cigarette smoking; possibly anorexia, weight loss, nausea, vomiting, weakness
Physical examination and diagnostic studies
• Possibly weight loss, consolidation, or atelectasis
• Possibly abnormal chest X-ray,

sputum cytology, bronchoscopy, and fiberoscopy

ADULT RESPIRATORY DISTRESS SYNDROME (ARDS)

Chief complaint
• *Cough:* dry, sputum progressing to rusty and frothy to burgundy red
• *Dyspnea:* tachypnea progressing to dyspnea
• *Chest pain:* absent
History
• Shock (septic, hemorrhagic, cardiogenic, anaphalactoid), direct chest trauma, aspiration, fat emboli, massive viral pneumonia
Physical examination and diagnostic studies
• Tachycardia; cyanosis; diffuse, scattered rales, progressing to poor respiratory excursion; normal fremitus; normal percussion; normal breath and voice sounds
• Chest X-ray abnormal; arterial blood gas analysis abnormal

ATELECTASIS

Chief complaint
• *Cough:* present
• *Dyspnea:* sudden; wheezing
• *Chest pain:* absent or pleuritic
History
• *Mild or chronic:* no signs or symptoms
• *Acute:* sudden signs or symptoms; recent surgery

Continued

Guide to Respiratory Disorders
Continued

ATELECTASIS
Continued

Physical examination and diagnostic studies
● Tachycardia; tracheal shift to affected side; respiratory excursion limited on affected side; tactile fremitus decreased or absent; dull-to-flat percussion over collapsed lung; hyperresonance over remaining portion of affected lung; decreased or absent breath and voice sounds; adventitious sounds high pitched with crackles, especially on inspiration
● Abnormal chest X-ray possible

Postoperative Hypoventilation: An Ounce of Prevention

A patient who's just out of surgery may find deep breathing painful or difficult. Unless you intervene, he could develop postoperative hypoventilation, a complication that can lead to atelectasis or pneumonitis. To encourage your patient to breathe normally, follow these guidelines:

Before surgery:
● Carefully evaluate the patient's history and clinical condition to detect factors that may predispose him to postoperative hypoventilation: lung disease, smoking, productive cough, shortness of breath, low exercise tolerance, heart disease or MI, or obesity.
Note: If the patient greatly risks postoperative hypoventilation, the doctor may want to place him in the ICU after surgery.

After surgery:
● Check with the doctor before administering drugs or increasing dosages of drugs that can cause respiratory depression.
● Provide emotional support. If your patient fears incision pain so much that he hesitates to move, try to allay his fears by explaining the importance of turning periodically. Establish a turning schedule for the patient to follow.
● Teach him proper techniques for deep breathing, coughing, and splinting. If he needs incentives spirometry exercises, teach him how to use the equipment (unless a respiratory therapist is available).

Classifying Acute Respiratory Failure (ARF)

Although ARF isn't itself a disease, it's a potential end result of many disease conditions—several of which may occur simultaneously. Conditions impairing ventilation initially produce hypercapnia; those impairing oxygenation produce hypoxemia. Read what follows for some common examples.

IMPAIRED VENTILATION

- Anaphylaxis
- Asthma
- Atelectasis
- Bronchitis
- Drug overdose (for example, of barbiturates or sedatives)
- Emphysema
- Fractures (especially of the ribs)
- Guillain-Barré syndrome
- Myasthenia gravis
- Pleural effusion
- Pneumonia
- Pneumothorax
- Thoracic surgery or trauma
- Upper airway obstruction (for example, by the tongue or a foreign body)

IMPAIRED OXYGENATION

- Adult respiratory distress syndrome (ARDS)
- Aspiration of acids or bile
- Lung tumors
- Near drowning
- Pulmonary emboli
- Pulmonary edema
- Toxic chemical inhalation

Respiratory Failure: Points to Remember

- Defining characteristics of acute respiratory failure usually include acute dyspnea, a PaO_2 less than 50 mm Hg, a $PaCO_2$ greater than 50 mm Hg, and acidosis.
- Recognition of high-risk patients is the key to early detection and successful treatment of respiratory failure.
- Four pathophysiologic mechanisms are responsible for impaired gas exchange: alveolar hypoventilation, ventilation/perfusion mismatch, intrapulmonary shunting, and impaired diffusion across the respiratory membrane
- The signs and symptoms of hypoxemia, hypercapnia, and acidosis are widespread, involving all major body systems.
- Oxygen therapy must be precisely controlled in hypercapnic respiratory failure to avoid dampening the patient's hypoxic drive to breathe.

Pathogenesis of ARF

Acute lung infection. Acute infection increases pulmonary secretions, causing atelectasis and increased work of breathing, which, in turn, causes ventilation/perfusion mismatch.

Heart failure or myocardial infarction. In heart failure and myocardial infarction, increased left ventricular end-diastolic volume causes blood to back up in the lungs, resulting in interstitial edema and decreased compliance. Increased work of breathing follows, triggering this cycle: increased work causes increased carbon dioxide production, which stimulates increased minute ventilation. Eventually, the lungs can't work hard enough to remove excess carbon dioxide, resulting in alveolar hypoventilation.

Pulmonary emboli. Pulmonary emboli may obstruct or impair blood flow to an area of alveoli, causing ventilation/perfusion mismatch.

Neuromuscular disorders. In neuromuscular disorders, weakening or paralysis of the muscles that control ventilation results in alveolar hypoventilation.

Respiratory depressants. Administration of respiratory depressants, such as sedatives, narcotics, and tranquilizers, causes alveolar hypoventilation. Injudicious administration of oxygen may also cause respiratory depression by dampening the patient's hypoxic drive to breathe.

Abdominal or thoracic injury or surgery. Shallow breathing due to incisional pain or administration of narcotics for pain relief causes respiratory depression and alveolar hypoventilation. Accumulation of secretions due to immobility and shallow breathing causes ventilation/perfusion mismatch. Ventilation/perfusion mismatching may also occur after pneumonectomy due to hyperperfusion of the remaining lung.

Special Consideration

A brief history from the patient or his family is indispensable to determine the cause of respiratory failure. Does the patient have a history of pulmonary disease? Has he recently aspirated any foreign material? Answers to such questions can separate acute respiratory failure from ARDS in chronic pulmonary disease—a crucial distinction for appropriate oxygen therapy.

Metabolic/Respiratory — Acidosis/Alkalosis: A Comparative Analysis

METABOLIC ACIDOSIS

Excess of acid (H^+) and deficit of base (HCO_3^-)
Probable cause: Ketoacidosis, diabetes, renal failure, diarrhea
Signs and symptoms: Headache, nausea, vomiting, diarrhea, sensorium changes, tremoring, convulsions
Laboratory tests: ph$<$7.35; serum $CO_2<$22 mEq/liter; $PaCO_2<$35 mm Hg if compensating; PaO_2 usually normal; serum potassium elevated

RESPIRATORY ACIDOSIS

Excess of carbonic acid (H_2CO_3) and elevated $PaCO_2$
Probable cause: Hypoventilation: retention of CO_2
Signs and symptoms: Decreased ventilation, sensorium changes, somnolence, semicomatose-comatose, tachycardia, dysrhythmia
Laboratory tests: pH$<$7.35; serum $CO_2>$26 mEq/liter if compensating; $PaCO_2>$ 45 mm Hg; PaO_2 usually normal or low; serum potassium elevated

METABOLIC ALKALOSIS

Deficit of acid (H^+) and excess of base (HCO_3^-)
Probable cause: Gastric losses via vomiting, stomach tube, lavage, potent diuretics
Signs and symptoms: Nausea, vomiting, diarrhea, sensorium changes, tremoring, convulsions
Laboratory tests: pH$>$7.45; serum $CO_2>$26 mEq/liter; $PaCO_2>$45 mm Hg if compensating; PaO_2 usually normal; serum potassium decreased; serum chloride decreased

RESPIRATORY ALKALOSIS

Deficit of carbonic acid (H_2CO_3) and decreased $PaCO_2$
Probable cause: Hyperventilation from neurogenic cause, brain trauma, ventilators
Signs and symptoms: Tachypnea, sensorium changes, numbness, tingling of hands and face
Laboratory tests: pH$>$7.45; serum $CO_2<$22 mEq/liter if compensating; $PaCO_2<$ 35 mm Hg; PaO_2 usually normal; serum potassium decreased; urine alkaline

Reviewing ARDS Care Priorities

When caring for a patient with adult respiratory distress syndrome (ARDS), put these goals at the top of your list:
• maintaining oxygenation and reducing oxygen consumption
• supporting oxygen transport
• sustaining cardiac output
• maintaining fluid and electrolyte balance.

To maintain oxygenation and reduce oxygen consumption
• Give oxygen as ordered.
• Promote bed rest, space activities, and decrease stressful stimuli.
• Maximize the patient's existing ventilations by having him cough and deep breathe every hour; performing nasopharyngeal suctioning, as needed; elevating the head of the bed to a comfortable position; and ensuring proper body alignment.
• Turn the patient frequently and use postural drainage with vibration and percussion to reduce mucus consolidation in lungs.
• Give bronchodilators, if ordered.
• Perform *passive* range-of-motion exercises.
• Control fever by checking the patient's temperature every 4 hours (or as needed); and give antipyretics, as ordered. Also use fever-reducing techniques: Remove excess clothing and blankets; apply an ice pack to patient's axilla, groin, and the back of his neck; and sponge him

with tepid water.
• Reduce pain by administering analgesics, as ordered, at the first sign of pain.

To support oxygen transport
• Monitor the patient's complete blood cell count. If the patient is anemic, administer packed cells as ordered.
• Assess peripheral circulation by noting pulses, temperatures, and color in limb. Also assess capillary refill time.

To sustain cardiac output
• Assess cardiovascular status regularly.
• Monitor hemodynamic readings and report any changes to the doctor.
• Observe the patient for signs of decreased cardiac output, including pallor, tachycardia, diaphoresis, and decreasing urine output.
• Administer adrenergic drugs, as ordered.
• Give volume expanders, as ordered.

To maintain fluid and electrolyte balance
• Monitor his fluid intake and output.
• Weigh him at the same time each day, using the same scale.
• Carefully monitor electrolyte values.
• Periodically inspect the patient for peripheral edema and listen for crackles, indicating fluid buildup.

Recognizing the Stages of ARDS

Many emergency conditions (for example, lung contusion, drug over-dose, or near drowning) can cause ARDS—adult respiratory distress syndrome. In turn, ARDS can lead to acute respiratory failure, itself an emergency.

You probably know what ARDS is: noncardiogenic pulmonary edema. But can you recognize ARDS when it's developing? This chart will help you recognize the six developmental stages of ARDS and intervene appropriately.

STAGES	SIGNS AND SYMPTOMS	NURSING INTERVENTIONS
1. Inflamed and damaged alveolar-capillary membrane	• Depend on underlying cause of ARDS	• Do a brief assessment. • Take the patient's vital signs. • Auscultate for abnormal breath sounds. • Prepare the patient for a chest X-ray. • Begin treatment of underlying cause to prevent further ARDS development.
2. Protein and water shift in the interstitial space	• Tachypnea, dyspnea, and tachycardia	• Draw blood for ABGs. • Prepare the patient for oxygen therapy, intubation, and mechanical ventilation. • Begin fluid management, avoiding fluid overload.
3. Pulmonary edema	• Increased tachypnea, dyspnea, and cyanosis • Hypoxemia (generally unresponsive to increased FIO_2) • Decreased pulmonary compliance • Rales and rhonchi	• Connect the patient to a mechanical ventilator with a positive end-expiratory pressure (PEEP) setting and a high oxygen concentration. • Watch for complications from ventilation therapy. *Continued*

Recognizing the Stages of ARDS
Continued

STAGES	SIGNS AND SYMPTOMS	NURSING INTERVENTIONS
4. Collapsed alveoli and impaired gas exchange	• Thick, frothy, sticky sputum • Marked hypoxemia with increased respiratory distress	• Anticipate that a Swan-Ganz catheter will be inserted to measure pulmonary capillary wedge pressure.
5. Decreased oxygen and carbon dioxide levels in the blood	• Increased tachypnea • Hypoxemia • Hypocapnia	• Study ABGs, mixed venous blood gases, and pulmonary capillary wedge pressure to understand the relationship between PEEP, intrapulmonary shunt, and cardiac output. • Monitor the patient's vital signs and urine output (hydration).
6. Hypoxemia; metabolic acidosis	• Decreased serum pH • Increased $PaCO_2$ level • Decreased PaO_2 level • Confusion • Decreased HCO_3^- level	• Watch for fluid restriction or overdiuresis that may cause hypovolemia, hypotension, and hypoperfusion. • Check for shock, coma, respiratory failure, and neurologic complications secondary to metabolic alterations and respiratory failure. • Reassure the patient and his family.

What Causes ARDS?

If you're like many nurses, you're a little confused about the exact cause of ARDS. Relax, your confusion is understandable. After all, ARDS is not a clearly defined disease. Instead, it's a possible complication of a variety of respiratory and nonrespiratory problems, including:
- shock
- septicemia (primarily gram-negative)
- trauma, such as a lung contusion, a head injury, or a long-bone fracture with a fat embolus
- viral, bacterial, or fungal pneumonia
- microemboli; for example, fat or air emboli
- disseminated intravascular coagulation (DIC)
- drug overdose
- aspiration of gastric contents
- smoke or chemical inhalation; for example, from nitrous oxide, chloride, or ammonia
- hydrocarbon or paraquat ingestion
- pancreatitis, uremia, or miliary tuberculosis (rare)
- near drowning
- fluid overload.

CONTROLLING RESPIRATORY DISORDERS

The Many Names of ARDS

If the signs and symptoms of ARDS sound familiar but the term "ARDS" doesn't, don't be surprised. Although ARDS is the commonly used term, its synonyms include:
- shock lung syndrome
- stiff lung syndrome
- adult hyaline membrane disease
- white lung
- wet lung
- Da Nang lung
- respiratory lung
- post pump lung
- acute pulmonary insufficiency
- acute ventilatory insufficiency
- posttraumatic pulmonary insufficiency
- noncardiogenic pulmonary edema
- hemorrhagic pulmonary edema
- post-nontraumatic pulmonary insufficiency.

Does Your Patient Have ARDS?

Have you already determined that your patient risks developing ARDS? If so, you'll want to be particularly alert for early clinical signs of it. By identifying ARDS early, you can improve his chances of recovery.

If you suspect ARDS, help confirm your suspicions by asking yourself these questions:
• Is the patient unusually restless, apprehensive, forgetful, or confused?
• Is he disoriented—even slightly? Is he exhibiting any unusual behavior; for example, mood shifts or inappropriate responses to others?
• Is he having difficulty breathing? If so, is he making a grunting sound or exhibiting increased chest movement on expiration?
• Are his pulse and temperature slightly elevated?
• Is he experiencing transient rises in arterial blood pressure?

• On lung auscultation, do you hear rales and rhonchi?
• If the patient is breathing room air, are his PaO_2 and $PaCO_2$ values dropping?
• If he's receiving oxygen therapy, are you giving higher oxygen concentrations without producing an increase in his PaO_2?
• If he's on a ventilator, is the amount of pressure needed to achieve a prescribed tidal volume increasing?
• Is he experiencing diaphoresis?
• Is his skin pale?

If you've answered *yes* to one or more of these questions, your patient may be developing ARDS. Notify the doctor immediately of your suspicions. To help confirm the diagnosis, he'll immediately order tests; for example, serial X-rays, and pulmonary artery pressure and pulmonary artery wedge pressure measurements. Expect to begin treatment at once.

Nursing Tip

Early clinical signs of ARDS are, at best, subtle. So, be on the lookout for conditions that may superficially parallel ARDS. These include:
• pulmonary edema from severe heart failure
• acute hypersensitivity lung disease
• fluid overload
• chronic interstitial fibrosis
• acute exacerbation of chronic lung disease

Monitoring Fluid Balance with PCWP

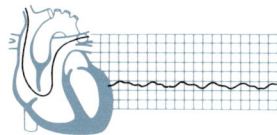

Using pulmonary capillary wedge pressure (PCWP) to evaluate fluid balance is fast becoming standard practice in the patient with ARDS—which comes as no surprise when you consider the potential dangers of fluid imbalance for this patient. For example, fluid overload may increase existing pulmonary edema, which may, in turn, increase intrapulmonary shunting and further decrease compliance. Underhydration may contribute to inadequate perfusion associated with ARDS or treatment with PEEP.

PCWP is obtained by threading a balloon-tipped, flow-directed catheter to the junction of the vena cava and right atrium. After inflation of the balloon, venous circulation carries the catheter tip through the right atrium and ventricle to a branch of the pulmonary artery, where the balloon wedges itself.

A PCWP above 12 mm Hg may indicate overhydration; below 6 mm Hg, underhydration. Monitoring this pressure guides fluid ther-

apy and, combined with the use of vasopressors, maintains balanced perfusion.

Inflating a PA catheter's balloon
You'll inflate the balloon at the end of the pulmonary artery (PA) catheter when you take a PCWP reading. In most cases, you'll inflate it with air. This is safe, even if the balloon ruptures, because the pulmonary artery will usually carry the escaping air bubbles to the lungs, where they're expelled.

Never use liquid to inflate the catheter's balloon. If you do, the balloon won't float properly or deflate completely.

Record the mean PCWP displayed on the monitor and immediately deflate the balloon. When the balloon's deflated, the catheter tip will float back into the main branch of the pulmonary artery.

In most cases, the doctor will not order PCWP readings to be taken more than once every 4 hours. More frequent inflations could rupture the balloon.

Important: Make sure the balloon's completely deflated at all times, except when you take a PCWP reading. Otherwise, the balloon may wedge in a branch of the pulmonary artery. And prolonged wedging, as you know, may cause a pulmonary infarction.

Near Drowning Signs and Symptoms

Check the victim for the following signs and symptoms of asphyxia and pulmonary edema:
• rapidly worsening dyspnea
• apnea
• wheezing and crackles
• productive cough with pink, frothy sputum
• substernal chest pain that worsens with breathing
• tachycardia
• vomiting
• abdominal distention
• cyanosis
• confusion, lethargy, irritability, or restlessness
• unconsciousness
• seizure
• coma
• elevated body temperature. (However, if the accident occurred in cold water, the patient's temperature may be abnormally low.)
• respiratory or cardiac arrest.

Helping the Near-Drowning Victim

You can begin cardiopulmonary resuscitation (CPR) as soon as the victim's head is above water. If you suspect a spinal injury, place a board under the victim's head and back while he's still in the water.

When the victim arrives at the hospital, your first priority is to maintain an open airway. Continue CPR, if necessary. Then take the following measures:
• Relieve hypoxemia. Administer low-percentage oxygen until you can obtain ABG measurements. Then ventilate the patient, as ordered, using intermittent positive pressure breathing (IPPB) with 100% oxygen or positive end-expiratory pressure (PEEP). Suction the patient's airway frequently to remove secretions.
• Monitor vital signs. Continue to do this even after the patient's condition has stabilized. Check his central venous pressure to assess cardiopulmonary status. Stay alert for signs of secondary drowning and increased respiratory distress (for example, confusion, chest pain, and adventitious breath sounds).
• Relieve abdominal distention. Insert a nasogastric tube and connect it to suction, as ordered.
• Administer appropriate medications. Be prepared to give isoproterenol to relieve bronchospasm; steroids to stabilize damaged capillary walls; and antibiotics to prevent infection.
• Monitor the patient's intake and output. Insert an indwelling (Foley) catheter and start an I.V. line to administer plasma.

Saltwater and Freshwater Aspiration: Two Routes to Hypoxia

Although the cause of death in drowning—and the ultimate danger in near drowning—is tissue hypoxia, the type of fluid aspirated determines how hypoxemia develops. Fresh water rapidly penetrates the pulmonary capillary membrane, causing alveolar collapse, intrapulmonary shunting, and hypoxemia.

Salt water disrupts osmotic pressure, forcing fluid into the alveoli. Pulmonary edema, intrapulmonary shunting, and hypoxemia result.

The chart below shows how fluid aspiration affects the body.

ARTERIAL BLOOD GASES

Effect
Hypoxemia

BLOOD VOLUME

Effect
Salt water: Persistent hypovolemia from hypertonic fluid entering the alveoli
Fresh water: Transient hypervolemia from rapid absorption of hypotonic fluid into the circulation

CARDIAC

Effect
Ventricular fibrillation from aspiration of large amounts of fluid (rare)

HEMOGLOBIN

Effect
Possible hemoglobin decrease; hemolysis after aspiration of 0.11 ml of fluid/kg of body weight

NEUROLOGIC

Effect
Altered mental status or coma from cerebral anoxia

SERUM ELECTROLYTES

Effect
Changes usually insignificant; severe hypoxemia and acidosis may cause hyperkalemia

URINARY

Effect
Acute renal failure from hypotension and hypoxemia

Risk Factors for Toxic Chemical Inhalation

As the use of synthetic materials increases, so does the risk of a chemical accident leading to toxic lung injury—a dangerous respiratory disorder resulting from toxic chemical inhalation. Workers or bystanders may suffer toxic chemical inhalation from an accident, such as a fire at a chemical plant.

Toxic lung injury can occur within minutes after exposure to noxious chemicals contained in smoke or gas. Without proper treatment, this injury can lead to respiratory failure.

Certain patients are more likely than others to sustain significant lung damage from toxic chemical inhalation. The following factors predispose a patient to serious lung damage:

• *Preexisting lung disease* that reduces ventilation, disturbs cell function, or destroys lung tissue; for example, tuberculosis, chronic obstructive pulmonary disease (COPD), or pleurisy. (Pulmonary edema is an exception. The excess fluid this condition produces helps mobilize harmful particles before they can irritate the alveolar wall.)

• *Cigarette smoking* paralyzes the mucociliary escalator—a system in which the cilia and a mucus blanket propel airway particles upward. This leads to bronchoconstriction and thick mucus buildup, which compromise the lungs' normal defense mechanisms by impairing macrophagic activity.

• *Long-term exposure to toxic chemicals* can wear out the lungs' defense mechanisms. (Most lung diseases take years to develop.)

• *Exposure to high concentrations of toxic chemicals,* even over a short period of time, may overwhelm the lungs' defense mechanisms.

• *The size of a chemical's particles* determines where those particles lodge in the lungs. For example, particles 3 to 5 microns in diameter lodge in the alveoli and cause the greatest amount of damage. Particles less than 1 micron in diameter (for example, those in smoke) cause less serious injury, since they penetrate the alveolar walls and enter interstitial tissue.

Toxic Chemical Inhalation: Assessment and Intervention

Do you suspect your patient's respiratory crisis was caused by toxic chemical inhalation? If you can answer yes to all or most of these questions, chances are he's inhaled a toxic chemical.

• Did the accident occur in a confined area? How long did the patient remain in the area?

• During the accident, did any synthetic materials burn? If so, which material was it? How much?

• Does he complain of a burning pain in his chest or throat?

• Are his upper airways mildly irritated?

• Are his nasal hairs singed?

• Does he have any facial burns?

• Is he restless or agitated?

• Do you detect rales or rhonchi on auscultation?

• Is he dyspneic?

• Is he wheezing, coughing, or hoarse?

• Is he hypoxemic?

• Does his sputum contain black carbon particles?

CONTROLLING RESPIRATORY DISORDERS

Nursing Tip

If your patient has inhaled toxic chemicals, take these nursing steps immediately:

• Assess and maintain his airway, breathing, and circulation. Initiate cardiopulmonary resuscitation if necessary.

• Administer low-percentage humidified oxygen until you can obtain ABG measurements.

• Assist with insertion of an endotracheal tube to improve breathing.

• As ordered, ventilate the patient using IPPB with 100% oxygen to enhance inspired oxygen and blood distribution and to improve the patient's ventilation/perfusion balance.

• Administer bronchodilators, as ordered.

• Give corticosteroids, if ordered.

• Insert a nasogastric tube to help remove ingested chemicals.

Later, after the patient's condition has stabilized, teach him to perform postural drainage, and encourage him to cough and deep breathe to help loosen and clear airway secretions.

Pathologic Responses to Smoke Inhalation

INITIAL RESPONSES

- Constriction of bronchioles
- Increased carboxyhemoglobin saturation
- Laryngeal edema
- Signs and symptoms: cough, cherry-red mucosa, stridor

DELAYED RESPONSES

- Increased pulmonary capillary permeability
- Destruction of lung parenchyma
- Signs and symptoms: dyspnea and crackles, increased sputum production, hyperinflation of lungs, rhonchi

Combating Carbon Monoxide Poisoning

Carbon monoxide poisoning, one of the most common poisoning types, accompanies most inhalation injuries. Colorless, odorless, and tasteless, carbon monoxide is found in acetylene gas, automobile exhaust, carbonyl iron, coal gas, furnace gas, illuminating gas, and marsh gas.

Assessment. To assess the severity of carbon monoxide poisoning, the doctor will order blood tests to determine the patient's carboxyhemoglobin level. Signs and symptoms of carbon monoxide poisoning vary in severity depending on the carboxyhemoglobin level. A level of 20% causes headache and mild dyspnea, whereas a level between 20% and 40% produces fatigue, irritability, diminished judgment, dimmed vision, and nausea.

When the carboxyhemoglobin level's between 40% and 60%, the patient suffers confusion, hallucinations, ataxia, collapse, and coma. His skin and mucous membranes turn cherry red.

Although ABG measurements may reveal a normal PaO_2 level, oxygen release to peripheral tissues drops sharply when carboxyhemoglobin levels are high.

Management. The doctor will order 100% high-flow oxygen, which reduces the half-life of carboxyhemoglobin from 4 hours to 30 minutes. He may order blood transfusions or hyperbaric oxygen therapy. This treatment provides 100% oxygen at high pressure in a controlled environment.

In addition to administering oxygen, keep the patient on total bed rest for at least 48 hours, or as ordered. Also watch for signs and symptoms of reduced cardiac output or central nervous system impairment, which may not appear until 3 weeks later.

COPD: Bronchial Airway Obstruction

The umbrella term *chronic obstructive pulmonary disease* (COPD) includes bronchitis, emphysema, and asthma. Although each condition has a distinctive pathophysiology, all are characterized by a narrowing of bronchial airways. By trapping air in the bronchioles and alveoli, this narrowing impairs ventilation, hinders gas exchange, and distends the alveoli.

Who's at risk. What causes COPD? The most important single predisposing factor is cigarette smoking; COPD is relatively rare in nonsmokers. Habitual smoking impairs ciliary action and macrophagic activity, causes airway inflammation and excessive mucus production, destroys alveolar septae, and encourages the development of peribronchiolar fibrosis. Prolonged exposure to irritating dust, fibers, and fumes—

COPD deaths
Deaths from COPD and related conditions totaled over 64,000 in 1983.

especially in combination with cigarette smoking—produces similar effects.

Other significant risk factors include the following:

● *Hereditary predisposition* contributes significantly to the development of asthma and—in some patients—emphysema. For example, an inherited deficiency of alpha$_1$-antitrypsin, a nonspecific proteolytic enzyme inhibitor, permits naturally occurring proteolytic enzymes to cause lung tissue lysis; this, in turn, leads to emphysema.

● *Aging* may be associated with mild panlobular emphysema, an often asymptomatic condition common among elderly patients.

● *Respiratory infection* is the primary cause of intrinsic (nonatopic) asthma. In addition, infections exacerbate all COPD types.

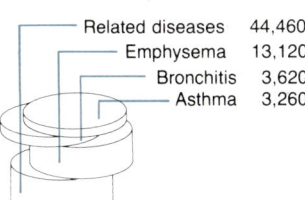

Related diseases	44,460
Emphysema	13,120
Bronchitis	3,620
Asthma	3,260

Effective Breathing Techniques

To help your patient prevent acute episodes of COPD, teach him to control his breathing by using either the abdominal or pursed-lip method. By practicing these methods regularly and using them during all his activities, he can keep his lungs free of stale air and gain confidence in managing his disorder.

   Use the instructions below as a teaching guide.

Abdominal breathing

Lie comfortably on your back, with your knees bent, and relax your abdomen.

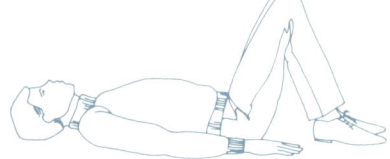

Next, press your hand (or place a book) lightly on your abdomen to create resistance.

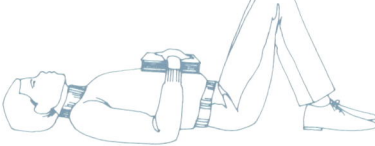

Keeping your chest still, begin breathing abdominally. You're performing the technique correctly if your abdomen and hands (or book) rise as you breathe in and fall as you breathe out.

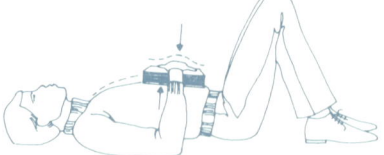

Continued

Effective Breathing Techniques
Continued

Pursed-lip breathing
Close your mouth and breathe in through your nose, taking a normal breath. (If you take too large a breath, you'll have to exhale much more air.)

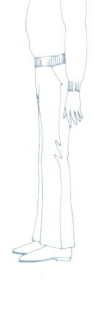

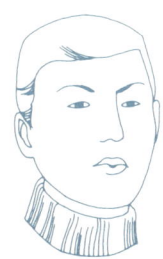

Now purse your lips as you would to whistle, and breathe out slowly through your mouth, without puffing your cheeks. Take at least twice the time you took to breathe in. Use your abdominal muscles to squeeze out every last bit of air you can.

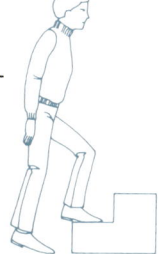

During physical activity, always inhale before exerting yourself; exhale while performing the activity. For example, when walking up stairs, inhale between steps; exhale while climbing.

Recognizing Acute Parenchymal Disease

INFLUENZA

Onset
Insidious
Early signs and symptoms
Low fever, malaise, headache, and, possibly, nonproductive cough
Late signs and symptoms
High fever, anorexia, persistent cough
Complicating disorders and diagnostic difficulties
Secondary bacterial or viral pneumonia may follow.

ACUTE BRONCHITIS

Onset
Insidious (develops as complication of other pulmonary illness)
Early signs and symptoms
Chest tightness; wheezing; hacking, productive cough; purulent, blood-tinged sputum
Late signs and symptoms
Fever, cyanosis, dyspnea

BACTERIAL PNEUMONIA

Onset
Abrupt
Early signs and symptoms
High fever; shaking, chills; pleuritic pain; productive cough with purulent, rusty sputum; hyperventilation; fever blisters

Late signs and symptoms
Increased severity of early symptoms
Complicating disorders and diagnostic difficulties
May present first as upper respiratory infection, with minor symptoms for a week.

VIRAL PNEUMONIA

Onset
Insidious
Early signs and symptoms
Cold or influenza symptoms: fever, malaise, nonproductive cough
Late signs and symptoms
High fever, dyspnea, purulent cough, blood-streaked sputum, cyanosis, respiratory failure
Complicating disorders and diagnostic difficulties
Localized form produces fewer symptoms. Diffuse form may produce severe symptoms and be complicated by bacterial pneumonia.

ASPIRATION PNEUMONIA

Onset
Insidious (latent period before onset, except in aspiration of large amounts of gastric juice or hydrocarbons)

Continued

Recognizing Acute Parenchymal Disease
Continued

ASPIRATION PNEUMONIA
Continued

Early signs and symptoms
Productive cough, perhaps containing gastric juice or food particles
Late signs and symptoms
Hemoptysis, copious secretions, superimposed bacterial pneumonia
Complicating disorders and diagnostic difficulties
Chronic aspiration may be asymptomatic until abscess formation.

LUNG ABSCESS

Onset
Insidious (symptoms of superimposed disease, such as bacterial infection, may be present)
Early signs and symptoms
Malaise, low-grade fever, chills, mild pleuritic pain
Late signs and symptoms
High fever, pleurisy, dyspnea, cyanosis, purulent cough when abscess drains
Complicating disorders and diagnostic difficulties
May be mistaken for pneumonia until abscess drains.

Treatment of Acute Parenchymal Disease

Bed rest and adequate fluid intake are key measures for treating influenza. Fluid replacement corrects loss of body fluids from fever and rapid breathing. Adequate fluid balance also loosens secretions, facilitating their removal through coughing. An expectorant helps relieve nonproductive coughing, and aspirin relieves fever and muscle pain.

In pneumonia, adequate fluid intake is important to maintain perfusion of vital organs and to reduce the heart's work load brought on by hypoxemia. If anemia is present, transfusion of whole blood may be needed to en-

Continued

Treatment of Acute Parenchymal Disease
Continued

hance the blood's oxygen-carrying capacity. Analgesics are usually needed to relieve pleuritic pain, which may be severe enough to require a narcotic such as morphine.

Administration of humidified oxygen aims to correct hypoxemia. Low flow rates of 4 to 6 liters per minute by nasal cannula or of 40% oxygen by mask usually restore adequate oxygenation. If hypoxemia is unresponsive to oxygen delivered by nasal cannula or mask (common in severe pneumonia), ventilator therapy with positive end-expiratory pressure (PEEP) is necessary. PEEP increases the alveolar surface area and helps open collapsed alveoli, thereby improving gas exchange.

Administer bronchodilators to decrease inflammation and prevent bronchospasm. Turn the patient every 2 hours to promote lung expansion. Before sleep, elevate the patient's head with two or three pillows to facilitate breathing. If the patient's on bed rest, perform or encourage leg exercises to reduce the risk of thrombophlebitis. Encourage early ambulation to promote lung expansion and help mobilize secretions.

Antimicrobial therapy varies with the causative pathogen and typically begins directly after collection of sputum samples, before culture results are known.

Unfortunately, viral pneumonias don't respond to antibiotic therapy. But if bacterial infection is superimposed, erythromycin or tetracycline may relieve some symptoms.

Similarly, aspiration pneumonia doesn't respond to antibiotic therapy unless the aspirate contained bacteria. Then, penicillin or other antimicrobial drugs may prove helpful, depending on the pathogen. Administration of high-dose steroids, a controversial therapy, may help minimize lung damage when instituted within 24 hours of aspiration. Other supportive measures include airway management and chest physiotherapy with postural drainage.

Differential Diagnosis of Acute Parenchymal Disease

BACTERIAL PNEUMONIA

History
Often preceded by viral infection, such as influenza; concomitant family or community involvement is rare due to long incubation period (up to 14 days); pleuritic chest pain

Physical exam
Localized, bronchial breath sounds; dullness on percussion; impaired chest movement due to pleuritic pain

Chest X-ray
Localized, well-defined hazy shadow; airspace consolidation

White blood cell (WBC) count
Elevated, usually above 15,000 mm³

Sputum culture and sensitivity
Abundant bacteria and WBCs

Blood culture
Positive in 25% to 40% of cases

Serologic tests
Not significant

POSTINFLUENZA VIRAL PNEUMONIA

History
Epidemic or family involvement common because of short incubation period and highly contagious infection

Physical exam
Minimal signs at influenza stage, uniformly decreased breath sounds and crepitus at pneumonia stage

Chest X-ray
May be negative initially; as disease progresses, diffuse, patchy consolidation appears, followed by the "white lung" appearance of ARDS in severe cases

White blood cell (WBC) count
Normal

Sputum culture and sensitivity
No bacteria, some epithelial debris, few WBCs

Blood culture
Negative

Serologic tests
Increased viral antibody titers

ASPIRATION PNEUMONIA

History
Recent vomiting after anesthesia, recent dental or mouth infection, or history of chronic alcoholism or neurologic disorder; bronchospasm, pleuritic chest pain

Physical exam
Decreased breath sounds over affected area

Chest X-ray
Small-volume aspiration resembles bacterial pneumonia; large-

Continued

Differential Diagnosis of Acute Parenchymal Disease
Continued

ASPIRATION PNEUMONIA
Continued

volume aspiration may produce diffuse atelectasis, pulmonary edema, and massive consolidation
White blood cell (WBC) count
Elevated in aspiration of oral secretions with anaerobic bacteria

Sputum culture and sensitivity
Gram-negative bacilli with anaerobic and aerobic bacteria
Blood culture
Negative
Serologic tests
Not significant

Health Teaching in Acute Parenchymal Disease

Of the many nursing goals in acute parenchymal disease, health teaching is one of the most important—and its success requires knowledge, skill, and patience. First, select an appropriate time for health teaching. Don't approach the anxious, dyspneic patient; the patient who's concerned about his next breath won't be receptive. Instead, wait until the patient is relaxed and comfortable, and encourage his family to be present.

Once you've established the appropriate climate for health teaching, consider the patient's cognitive ability and use terms he can readily understand. Explain the symptoms and effects of respiratory infection and measures to control them. Review the signs and symptoms of early infection—cough, sore throat, fever—that re-

quire immediate medical attention. Carefully outline discharge instructions, including activity and dietary restrictions and the drug regimen. Be sure the patient understands the dosage, route, schedule, and side effects of prescribed drugs. If appropriate, encourage the patient to stop smoking. Describe environmental factors that aggravate or cause respiratory infection. Emphasize the importance of adequate indoor ventilation and of avoiding areas of high air pollution. Document your teaching and the patient's response.

Consider your interventions effective if the patient and his family understand the disease, reportable signs and symptoms, drug regimen, and environmental hazards.

Comparing Types of Pneumonia

VIRAL
INFLUENZA

(prognosis poor even with treatment; 50% mortality)
Signs and symptoms
• Cough (initially nonproductive; later, purulent sputum), marked cyanosis, dyspnea, high fever, chills, substernal pain and discomfort, moist rales, frontal headache, and myalgia
• Death results from cardiopulmonary collapse.
Diagnosis
• *Chest X-ray:* diffuse bilateral bronchopneumonia radiating from hilus
• *WBC:* normal to slightly elevated
• *Sputum smears:* no specific organisms
Treatment
Supportive: for respiratory failure, endotracheal intubation and ventilator assistance; for fever, hypothermia blanket or antipyretics; for influenza A, amantadine

ADENOVIRUS

(insidious onset; generally affects young adults)
Signs and symptoms
• Sore throat, fever, cough, chills, malaise, small amounts of mucoid sputum, retrosternal chest pain, anorexia, rhinitis, adenopathy, scattered rales, and rhonchi
Diagnosis
• *Chest X-ray:* patchy distribution of pneumonia, more severe than indicated by physical examination
• *WBC:* normal to slightly elevated
Treatment
• Treat symptoms only.
• Mortality low; usually clears with no residual effects

RESPIRATORY SYNCYTIAL VIRUS (RSV)

(most prevalent in infants and children)
Signs and symptoms
• Listlessness, irritability, tachypnea with retraction of intercostal muscles, slight sputum production, fine moist rales, fever, severe malaise, and, possibly, cough or croup
Diagnosis
• *Chest X-ray:* patchy bilateral consolidation
• *WBC:* normal to slightly elevated
Treatment
• *Supportive:* humidified air, oxygen, antimicrobials often given until viral etiology confirmed
• Complete recovery in 1 to 3 weeks

Continued

Comparing Types of Pneumonia
Continued

MEASLES/RUBEOLA

Signs and symptoms
• Fever, dyspnea, cough, small amounts of sputum, coryza, skin rash, and cervical adenopathy
Diagnosis
• *Chest X-ray:* reticular infiltrates, sometimes with hilar lymph node enlargement
• *Lung tissue specimen:* characteristic giant cells
Treatment
• *Supportive:* bed rest, adequate hydration, antimicrobials; assisted ventilation, if necessary

CHICKENPOX/VARICELLA

(uncommon in children, but present in 30% of adults with varicella)
Signs and symptoms
• Cough, dyspnea, cyanosis, tachypnea, pleuritic chest pain, hemoptysis and rhonchi 1 to 6 days after onset of rash
Diagnosis
• *Chest X-ray:* shows more extensive pneumonia than indicated by physical examination, and bilateral, patchy, diffuse, nodular infiltrates
• *Sputum analysis:* predominant mononuclear cells and characteristic intranuclear inclusion bodies, with characteristic skin rash, confirm diagnosis

Treatment
• *Supportive:* adequate hydration and oxygen therapy

CYTOMEGALOVIRUS(CMV)

Signs and symptoms
• Difficult to distinguish from other nonbacterial pneumonias
• Fever, cough, shaking chills, dyspnea, cyanosis, weakness, and diffuse rales
• Occurs in neonates as devastating multisystemic infection; in normal adults resembles mononucleosis; in immunocompromised hosts, varies from clinically inapparent to devastating infection
Diagnosis
• *Chest X-ray:* in early stages, variable patchy infiltrates; later, bilateral, nodular, and more predominant in lower lobes
• *Percutaneous aspiration of lung tissue, transbronchial biopsy, or open lung biopsy:* microscopic examination shows typical intranuclear and cytoplasmic inclusions; the virus can be cultured from lung tissue
Treatment
• Generally, benign and self-limiting in mononucleosis-like form
• *Supportive:* adequate hydration and nutrition, oxygen therapy, bed rest
• In immunosuppressed patients, disease is severe, even fatal.
Continued

Comparing Types of Pneumonia
Continued

BACTERIAL
STREPTOCOCCUS

(Diplococcus pneumoniae)
Signs and symptoms
● Sudden onset of a single, shaking chill, and sustained temperature of 102° to 104° F. (38.9° to 40° C.); often preceded by upper respiratory tract infection
Diagnosis
● *Chest X-ray:* areas of consolidation, often lobar
● *WBC:* elevated
● *Sputum culture:* may show gram-positive *S. pneumoniae;* this organism not always recovered
Treatment
● *Antimicrobial therapy:* penicillin G or a cephalosporin for 7 to 10 days. Such therapy begins after obtaining culture specimen but without waiting for results.

KLEBSIELLA

Signs and symptoms
● Fever and recurrent chills; cough producing rusty, bloody, viscous sputum (currant jelly); cyanosis of lips and nail beds due to hypoxemia; shallow, grunting respirations
● Likely in patients with chronic alcoholism, pulmonary disease, and diabetes

Diagnosis
● *Chest X-ray:* typically, but not always, consolidation in the upper lobe that causes bulging of fissures
● *WBC:* elevated
● *Sputum culture and Gram stain:* may show gram-positive cocci *Klebsiella*
Treatment
● *Antimicrobial therapy:* gentamicin, tobramycin, kanamycin, or a cephalosporin

STAPHYLOCOCCUS

Signs and symptoms
● Temperature of 102° to 104° F. (38.9° to 40° C.), recurrent shaking chills, bloody sputum, dyspnea, tachypnea, and hypoxemia
● Should be suspected with viral illness, such as influenza or measles, and in patients with cystic fibrosis
Diagnosis
● *Chest X-ray:* multiple abscesses and infiltrates; high incidence of empyema
● *WBC:* elevated
● *Sputum culture and Gram stain:* may show gram-positive staphylococci
Treatment
● *Antimicrobial therapy:* nafcillin or oxacillin for 14 days
● Chest tube drainage of empyema

Continued

Comparing Types of Pneumonia
Continued

ASPIRATION

Results from vomiting and aspiration of gastric or oropharyngeal contents into trachea and lungs.
Signs and symptoms
• Noncardiogenic pulmonary edema may follow damage to respiratory epithelium from contact with stomach acid.
• Crackles, dyspnea, cyanosis, hypotension, and tachycardia
• May be subacute pneumonia

with cavity formation, or lung abscess may occur if foreign body is present
Diagnosis
• *Chest X-ray:* locates areas of infiltrates, which suggest diagnosis
Treatment
• *Antimicrobial therapy:* penicillin G or clindamycin
• *Supportive:* oxygen therapy, suctioning, coughing, deep breathing, adequate hydration, and I.V. steroids

Formulating a Nursing Diagnosis: Begin with the Interview

For valuable information about the onset, duration, and characteristics of parenchymal infection, ask the patient with suspected bacterial or viral pneumonia these questions:
• Did your illness begin with symptoms of influenza—malaise, low fever, headache, or nonproductive cough? Do any family members have similar symptoms?

• How many windows are in your home? Is there good cross ventilation? How many people live in your home? Then focus on the patient's workplace. Is it poorly ventilated or overcrowded?
• Do you smoke? If so, for how long and how much?
• Do you have a history of chronic lung disease? If so, when were you last hospitalized?

Continued

Formulating a Nursing Diagnosis: Begin with the Interview

Continued

Ask the patient with suspected aspiration pneumonia these questions:
• Have you had anesthesia recently? Have you had a recent oral or dental infection?
• Do you drink alcohol often? How much? Has it ever caused you to lose consciousness?

The patient's answers to these questions may pinpoint problem areas that will help you formulate nursing diagnoses. For example, the patient who lives or works in a poorly ventilated, crowded environment may not realize how this contributes to the spread of influenza. For this patient the nursing diagnosis—knowledge deficit related to disease—readily follows, with health teaching your appropriate intervention.

Fighting the Infection

After the doctor's identified the cause of your patient's pneumonia, he'll probably order one or a combination of several antimicrobial drugs. The doctor may also order an analgesic to relieve pleuritic pain and a bronchodilator to improve expectoration.

Also take these other supportive measures when caring for a patient with pneumonia:
• Maintain adequate fluid intake.
• Encourage the patient to eat a high-calorie diet.
• Administer humidified oxygen to correct hypoxemia (usually 4 to 6 liters/minute by nasal cannula or mask).

Note: If the patient's anemic, a blood transfusion may be ordered to restore oxygen-carrying capacity. If he has *severe* pneumonia, he'll probably be transferred to the intensive care unit for positive end-expiratory pressure (PEEP).

Diagnostic Tests for Lung Cancer

CHEST X-RAY

Purpose
Locate tumor, pneumonia, or pleural effusion (not diagnostic)

SPUTUM ANALYSIS

Purpose
Search for cancer cells to diagnose lung, head/neck cancer

BRONCHOSCOPY

Purpose
Locate central tumor and biopsy for tissue, brush and wash suspect area for peripheral tumor, diagnose cell type

COMPUTERIZED TOMOGRAPHY (CT SCAN)

Purpose
Locate tumor, determine extent of disease (not diagnostic), plan surgical strategy, determine radiation port

RADIONUCLIDE SCANS

Purpose
Determine extent of brain, liver, or bone metastasis and adrenal gland involvement after confirmed diagnosis

MEDIASTINOSCOPY

Purpose
Diagnose metastasis from right lung or left lower lobe tumor, determine operability

MEDIASTINOTOMY

Purpose
Diagnose metastasis from left upper lobe or left hilar tumor, determine operability

THORACENTESIS

Purpose
Diagnose pleural effusion, determine operability

NEEDLE BIOPSY OF PLEURA

Purpose
Diagnose tumor involvement of pleura

NEEDLE BIOPSY OF TUMOR

Purpose
Diagnose tumor in selected cases

THORACOTOMY

Purpose
Diagnose tumor when other methods fail or in selected patients with peripheral nodules

Lung Cancer Prognosis by Cell Type

CHARACTERISTIC/ EPIDERMOID (SQUAMOUS)	ADENO- CARCINOMA	LARGE-CELL	SMALL-CELL
Approximate incidence/ 25% to 30%	30% to 35%	15% to 20%	20% to 25%
5-year survival/ 16% to 18%	10% to 12%	10% to 12%	4%
Operability/ 43% to 50%	35%	35% to 43%	Rare
Doubling time: mean/range (days)/88 days; 7 to 381 days	161 days 17 to 590 days	92 days 48 to 112 days	29 days 17 to 71 days
Potential for metastasis/ Low to moderate	Moderate	Moderate	High
Location in lung field/Central	Peripheral	Peripheral	Central
Response rate to systemic treatment/Low	Low	Low	Moderate

Recognizing Signs and Symptoms of Pleural Effusion

A patient with pleural effusion may complain of various signs and symptoms. The most common complaint is chest pain so severe that he fears he's having a heart attack. Such pain may even give rise to other symptoms, depending on the effusion's extent and the patient's pulmonary status. Signs and symptoms to watch for are listed here:

• dyspnea; may indicate minimal lung collapse
• sharp, stabbing chest pain aggravated by coughing or deep breathing (such as during exertion); relieved by short, shallow breaths and splinting; may radiate to neck, shoulders, or abdomen (since pain arises in intercostal nerves)
• shortness of breath (possibly from severe pain)
• dull or flat percussion, especially over the effusion
• absent or diminished voice sounds

• absent or diminished breath sounds over affected areas
• displaced heart sounds; may indicate mediastinal shift
• gallop heart rhythms; may indicate heart failure, frequently causing or accompanying effusion
• hypoxemia secondary to underlying respiration disorders or lung compression
• reduced lung volumes and areas of ventilation-perfusion mismatch.

Also check the patient's chart for any of the following factors that may predispose him to pleural effusion:
• preexisting fever, malaise, or purulent sputum
• a history of cardiac, hepatic, or renal disease
• recent drug therapy with hydralazine, methysergide, nitrofurantoin, or procainamide.

Nursing Tip

Advise the patient with pleural effusion to lie on the affected *side*, and show him how to splint the painful area when coughing or breathing deeply. Raise the head of his bed, or encourage him to sit up as much as possible. Both positions relax chest and abdominal muscles and make coughing less laborious.

Recognizing Signs and Symptoms of Pneumothorax

A patient with a small pneumothorax may not experience any signs or symptoms. A patient with a tension pneumothorax or a mild-to-moderate spontaneous or traumatic pneumothorax may have the following signs and symptoms:
• sudden, sharp pain on the affected side that increases with chest movement, coughing, and breathing and may radiate to the shoulder
• asymmetric chest wall movement
• shortness of breath
• anxiety
• subcutaneous emphysema in the neck and upper chest
• cyanosis
• rapid pulse and respiratory rate
• sucking sound near the wound
• neck vein distention.

History. A patient's chest pain and shortness of breath may cause you to confuse pneumothorax with myocardial ischemia, a dissecting aortic aneurysm, or pulmonary embolism. To help rule out these disorders, take a thorough history.

Physical examination.
Check for decreased or absent chest movement and breath sounds on the affected side. Auscultate for decreased or absent breath sounds over the collapsed lung. However, keep in mind that pain and splinting will affect these sounds.

Percuss for hyperresonance and decreased tactile fremitus on the affected side. Palpate for tracheal deviation to the unaffected side and crackling under the skin and for decreased vocal fremitus on the affected side.

Diagnostic tests. The doctor will probably order the following tests to confirm pneumothorax:
• *Chest X-ray.* This test will probably reveal a lowered diaphragm, air in the pleural cavity, chest wall expansion, and partial or total lung collapse on the affected side.
• *Arterial blood gases (ABGs).* These values usually show PaO_2 less than 80 mm Hg, $PaCO_2$ less than 35 mm Hg, and pH greater than 7.45, indicating hypoxemia and respiratory alkalosis.

Assessing Pulmonary Contusion

Signs and symptoms of pulmonary contusion are usually well-defined. You can classify most pulmonary contusions as mild, moderate, or severe, according to physical findings. For a convenient comparison of the signs and symptoms of pulmonary contusion types, study the chart below:

MILD PULMONARY CONTUSION

Signs and symptoms
- Chest pain
- Loose cough that produces copious and possibly blood-tinged secretions
- Tachypnea
- Tachycardia
- Loose crackles

MODERATE PULMONARY CONTUSION

Signs and symptoms
- Incessant cough that doesn't clear secretions
- Frank bleeding in the tracheobronchial tree
- Labored respirations
- Restlessness

- Apprehension
- Progressive respiratory insufficiency with dyspnea, tachypnea, and cyanosis

SEVERE PULMONARY CONTUSION

Signs and symptoms
- Incessant cough that produces copious amounts of frothy, blood-tinged secretions
- Agitation, restlessness, or combativeness
- Frank hemoptysis
- Rapid and labored respirations
- Wheezing and crackles
- Bronchial breath sounds
- Tachycardia
- Cyanosis

Special Consideration

Pulmonary contusion usually heals without surgery. While your patient's recovering, continue to maintain good pulmonary hygiene; monitor his respiratory status and vital signs frequently; and check his ABG results routinely.
- If you note hypoxemia and acidosis along with respiratory distress, tachycardia, fever, scattered crackles, and pink, frothy sputum, your patient may be developing adult respiratory distress syndrome (ARDS). Notify the doctor immediately. He will initiate aggressive ventilatory support, possibly including mechanical ventilation. The doctor will begin a program to wean him from the ventilator when his respiratory status is stabilized.

Assisting with Chest Tube Insertion

The doctor places a chest tube in your patient's pleural space to:
• drain air, blood, fluid, or pus from his pleural space
• reestablish atmospheric and intrathoracic pressure gradients
• allow complete lung reexpansion.

You may assist by reassuring the patient, preparing him for the procedure, and monitoring his recovery.

Indications
• Pneumothorax
• Hemothorax
• Empyema
• Pleural effusion
• Chylothorax

Complications
• Bleeding from intercostal blood vessels at insertion site
• Pulmonary laceration
• Tube placed into lung instead of pleural space
• Tension pneumothorax

Equipment
• Sterile gloves
• Betadine solution and prep sponges
• Sterile drapes
• Petrolatum gauze
• Dressing sponges and tape
• Local anesthetic, needles, syringes
• Chest tube tray that includes scalpel, assorted hemostats, curbed clamp (Kelly), trocar, chest tubes of assorted sizes
• Underwater-seal chest drainage system. (Your hospital may use the disposable Pleur-evac system, its equivalent three-bottle drainage system, or a one- or two-bottle water-seal system.)

Procedure
• Explain the procedure to the patient, indicating that this procedure will help him breathe more easily.
• Sedate him as ordered.
• Assist in preparing his skin with povidone-iodine solution.
• Drape the area with sterile towels.
• The doctor will anesthetize the skin area where he plans to insert the tube.
• Help the patient hold still while the doctor makes a skin incision and inserts the tube.
• To relieve *pneumothorax*, the doctor will insert the chest tube in the second intercostal space along the midclavicular line. For *pleural effusion* or *hemothorax*, he'll insert it in the fourth to sixth intercostal space in the anterior or midaxillary line.
• Connect the tube to the Pleur-evac underwater-seal chest drainage system.
• The doctor will suture the tube in place and apply petrolatum gauze and a sterile dressing.

Continued

Assisting with Chest Tube Insertion
Continued

• Tape all tube connections securely and regulate suction as ordered.
• Secure the Pleur-evac system to the patient's bed.

Nursing follow-up care
• Prepare the patient for a chest X-ray to check tube placement.
• Administer pain medication as ordered.
• Secure the tube to the draw sheet with a safety pin, allowing sufficient tubing for the patient to turn over. Don't leave dangling loops.

• Keep clamps and extra petrolatum gauze at the patient's bedside in case the tubing accidentally disconnects or pulls out.
• Watch for signs of chest tube occlusion from kinks, clots, or mucous plugs.
• Record hourly drainage on the collection chamber of the Pleur-evac.
• Observe the suction chamber for continuous bubbling. Lack of bubbling may indicate suction failure.

Nursing Tip

If your patient's chest tube gets accidentally disconnected from the drainage tube, reconnect it immediately. If you can't because you've lost or broken a connector, clamp the chest tube until you've remedied the problem. Work quickly so you can reconnect the tube as soon as possible. Remember to unclamp the chest tube when you've completed the connection.

If your patient's chest tube falls out or is accidentally pulled out, quickly seal off the insertion site to prevent air from entering his pleural cavity. Use petrolatum gauze and cover it with 4″ × 4″ gauze pads. Tape securely. If gauze isn't handy, temporarily seal the insertion site with a folded towel. Call the doctor immediately. Ask another nurse to get the equipment the doctor will need to reinsert the tubes.

Don't leave the patient. Watch him for signs of pneumothorax. Tension pneumothorax may occur because you've sealed off the only escape route for accumulating air or fluid. If danger signs do appear, remove the dressings immediately.

Monitoring Chest Drainage Systems

• Look for fluid fluctuation of 2″ to 4″ (5 to 10 cm) in the water-seal straw or chamber as the patient breathes. With mechanical suction, fluctuation is minimal; with positive-pressure ventilation, the usual direction of fluctuation (inspiratory rise, expiratory fall) reverses. Fluctuation stops with tube obstruction, faulty suction, or lung reexpansion.

• Observe for intermittent bubbling in the water-seal bottle or chamber during expiration. Absence of bubbling indicates that evacuation is complete and pressure of the expanded lung has sealed the chest tube opening. Constant bubbling indicates a leak.

• Look for gentle bubbling in the suction control bottle or chamber, indicating a proper suction level. Vigorous bubbling increases the water evaporation rate.

• Check air vent patency. Occlusion increases pressure and can lead to tension pneumothorax.

• Milk the tubing as needed to keep it patent. Perform this procedure cautiously, since the temporary rebound pressure when tubing is released can exceed -400 cmH_2O (normal intrapleural pressure is -5 cmH_2O) and may cause tissue damage. Also, the average patient may not need it, as blood remaining in the pleural space for a few hours rarely clots, and serous drainage rarely causes obstruction.

• Clamp the tubing only to locate the source of a leak or to replace a full or cracked collection bottle. Then clamp it only momentarily, since clamping halts air and fluid evacuation from the pleural space and can lead to tension pneumothorax. Preferable methods for changing bottles include having the able patient perform Valsalva's maneuver; and temporarily holding the tube's drainage end under water, sterile saline solution, or I.V. solution.

Special Consideration

Observe the amount, color, and consistency of chest drainage by looking through the plastic connector between the chest tube and the drainage tube. Check it hourly for the first 24 hours after chest tube insertion; then once every 2 hours. Document your findings.

At no time should bloody drainage exceed 100 ml per hour. If it does, notify the doctor at once.

Keep the label on the drainage bottle up to date. Write the amount of drainage that your patient's had over an 8-hour shift.

Managing a Sucking Chest Wound

If a sharp object or fragment from a missile injury penetrated your patient's chest wall, it may have created a sucking chest wound. Such a wound destroys the necessary pressure gradient between the pleural space and outside atmosphere. Unless you can restore this pressure gradient, the patient will quickly develop respiratory failure.

Equipment
● Nasal cannula, face masks, oxygen equipment
● Petrolatum gauze
● Wide tape
● Chest tube tray
Procedure
● Monitor your patient closely.
● Administer oxygen through a nasal cannula or a face mask.
● Don't remove any object protruding from your patient's chest-doing so will destroy the pressure gradient even faster and increase bleeding.
● Reassure the patient, then ask him to exhale forcefully. At the moment of maximum expiration, cover the wound with petrolatum gauze to seal it.
● Secure the gauze with wide tape.
● Monitor the patient closely for signs and symptoms of tension pneumothorax, and notify the doctor if this condition develops.
● If the doctor decides to insert a chest tube, get the equipment ready and be prepared to assist.

Assessing a Patient with a Penetrating Wound

Before examining a patient with a penetrating wound, first evaluate his ABC's. Then obtain as much information as possible from him about the incident. If he's unconscious or disoriented, question a family member, friend, or medical personnel, or speak to any police officers who were at the crime scene.

Since any gunshot or stabbing injury must be reported to the proper authorities, any information may be important legally. Make sure your documentation is thorough and accurate.

Guide to Acute Respiratory Disorders

You'll probably encounter patients with acute respiratory disorders more than patients with any other type of condition.

To refresh your memory of various types of acute respiratory disorders and your role in caring for these patients, read the following chart.

CROUP

Severe inflammation and obstruction of the upper airway; may be mistaken for and usually follows upper respiratory tract infection; more common in children. Three types exist: acute laryngotracheobronchitis, laryngitis, and acute spasmodic laryngitis.

Signs and symptoms
• Inspiratory stridor
• Hoarse or muffled sounds
• Sharp, barklike cough
• Inflammatory edema and possibly spasm, which may obstruct airway and compromise ventilation
For laryngotracheobronchitis:
• Fever
• Edema of the bronchi and bronchioles
• Expiratory rhonchi
• Scattered rales
For laryngitis:
• Sore throat and cough, possibly progressing to marked hoarseness
For acute spasmodic laryngitis:
• Mild-to-moderate hoarseness and nasal discharge, followed by cough and noisy inspiration
• Labored breathing with retractions, rapid pulse, clammy skin

• Suprasternal and intercostal retractions, dyspnea, diminished breath sounds, restlessness
Nursing interventions
• Promote bed rest.
• Administer aspirin or acetaminophen in recommended dosages.
• Obtain throat specimen for culture to help identify infecting organism (if bacteria's the cause).
• Urge use of cool-mist humidifier during sleep.
• Instruct parents to monitor cough and breath sounds, hoarseness, cyanosis, respiratory rate and character, restlessness, and fever.
• To relieve a croup spell, tell parents to carry child into the bathroom, shut the door, and turn on the hot water.
• To help control coughing, encourage parents to position two or three pillows under the child's head.
• Warn parents that ear infection and pneumonia are complications of croup that may appear within 5 days after recovery. Tell them to watch for and immediately report earache, productive cough, high fever, or increased shortness of breath.

Continued

Guide to Acute Respiratory Disorders
Continued

ACUTE BACTERIAL SINUSITIS

Inflammation of the paranasal sinus mucosa; recurrence may lead to chronic condition
Signs and symptoms
• Nasal congestion, followed by gradual buildup of pressure in the affected sinus
• Possibly purulent nasal discharge
• Low-grade fever
• Sore throat
• Malaise
• Pain and swelling over the affected sinus
Nursing interventions
• Stress to your patient the importance of taking the antibiotic medication ordered by the doctor.
• Advise your patient to take an oral antihistamine-decongestant combined with aspirin or acetaminophen.
• Teach your patient how to use nasal decongestant spray correctly.
• Encourage fluid intake to mobilize secretions and promote drainage.
• Tell your patient to watch for and report any of the following signs and symptoms of complications: vomiting, chills, fever, edema of forehead or eyelids, blurred or double vision, or personality changes.

BRONCHITIS

Inflammation of the tracheobronchial tree; more common in adults, especially those with chronic lung disease
Signs and symptoms
• Cough; may or may not be productive
• Coarse rhonchi or wheezes on lung auscultation
• Nasal discharge
• Fever
• Malaise
Nursing interventions
• Promote bed rest.
• Administer aspirin or acetaminophen in recommended dosages.
• Urge patient to take all the antibiotic medicine prescribed by the doctor, if appropriate.
• Recommend use of cool-mist vaporizer to help loosen secretions.
• Tell patient to use cough medicine with an expectorant to remove secretions.

INFLUENZA

Acute, highly contagious respiratory tract infection; occurs sporadically or in epidemics, especially during winter
Signs and symptoms
• Fever
• Malaise

Continued

Guide to Acute Respiratory Disorders
Continued

INFLUENZA *Continued*

- Myalgia
- Headache
- Sore throat
- Sudden onset of chills
- Cough

Nursing interventions
- Promote bed rest.
- Suggest increased fluid intake.
- Administer aspirin or acetaminophen in recommended dosages.
- Administer cough medicine with an expectorant.
- If signs and symptoms persist, instruct patient to return to the doctor for further evaluation.

NASOPHARYNGITIS

Infection causing mucosal edema and vasodilation

Signs and symptoms
- Possibly fever, especially in infants and young children
- Dry, irritated nose and throat, possibly accompanied by sneezing and coughing
- Irritability and restlessness
- Chills
- Muscle soreness

Nursing interventions
- Promote bed rest.
- Administer aspirin or acetaminophen in recommended dosages.
- If ordered, obtain a throat specimen for culture to test for streptococcal infection.

- Encourage increased fluid intake.
- Teach patient how to use nose drops to relieve nasal congestion.

PHARYNGITIS

Acute or chronic inflammation of the pharynx; usually lasts 3 to 10 days; most common throat disorder.

Signs and symptoms
- Sore throat
- Difficulty swallowing
- Sensation of lump in throat
- Constant urge to swallow
- On physical exam, posterior wall of pharynx appears red and edematous; mucous membranes studded with white or yellow follicles
- Exudate, usually confined to lymphoid areas
- May be accompanied by mild fever, headache, and muscle and joint pain (especially if bacteria's the cause)

Nursing interventions
- Obtain throat specimen or culture to identify causative organism.
- Promote bed rest.
- Administer aspirin or acetaminophen in recommended dosages.
- Teach patient with chronic pharyngitis how to minimize throat irritation; for example, by using a humidifier while sleeping.

Continued

Guide to Acute Respiratory Disorders
Continued

PHARYNGITIS
Continued

• Tell your patient to gargle with warm salt water to relieve sore throat pain.
• Administer throat lozenges containing a mild anesthetic.
• Encourage increased fluid intake.
• Administer penicillin, as ordered (if bacteria's the cause).

TONSILLITIS

Inflammation of the tonsils; may be acute or chronic; acute form usually lasts 4 to 6 days and commonly affects children between ages 5 and 10.
Signs and symptoms
For acute tonsillitis:
• Mild-to-severe sore throat
• Loss of appetite (in young child)
• Dysphagia
• Fever
• Chills
• Swelling and tenderness of lymph glands in submandibular area
• Muscle and joint pain
• Malaise
• Headache
• Possibly earache
• Generalized inflammation of pharyngeal wall

• Possibly edematous and inflamed uvula
• Swollen tonsils with white or yellow exudate
For chronic tonsillitis:
• Recurrent sore throat
• Purulent drainage in tonsillar crypts
• Frequent attacks of acute tonsillitis
• Peritonsillar abscess
Nursing interventions
• Administer aspirin or acetaminophen in recommended dosages.
• Administer antibiotics, as ordered (if bacteria's the cause).
• Obtain throat specimen for culture to determine infecting organism and appropriate antibiotic therapy (if bacteria's the cause).
• Suggest gargling to soothe the throat, unless it exacerbates the pain.
• Make sure the patient and parents understand the importance of completing prescribed course of antibiotic therapy.
• Encourage increased fluid intake.
• Promote bed rest.
• Suggest that parents give child ice cream or flavored drinks and ices.
• If tonsil removal is necessary, explain the procedure.

Guide to Occupational Lung Disorders

DISORDER/HIGH-RISK OCCUPATIONS	PATIENT HISTORY
Silicosis/Miners (lead, hard coal, copper, silver, and gold), foundry workers, potters, and sandstone and granite cutters	Exposure to free silica
Coal worker's pneumoconiosis (black lung disease)/Coal miners	Long-term exposure to coal dust in conjunction with excessive cigarette smoking
Berylliosis (beryllium disease, Wegener's granulomatosis)/Workers in chemical, military, ceramic, and aerospace industries who have contact with beryllium	Exposure to dust or fumes containing beryllium or its compounds, including sulfate and halide salts and beryllium oxide
Asbestosis/Workers involved in the mining, milling, manufacturing, or application of asbestos products, such as brake linings or insulation	Exposure to asbestos
Occupational asthma/Workers in cotton, leather, beer, wood, detergent, flax, and hemp industries (list is continually growing)	Exposure to irritants or allergenic particles or vapors
Acute chemical exposure/Workers who handle chlorine, phosgene, sulfur dioxide, hydrogen sulfide, nitrogen dioxide, and ammonia gases	Excessive exposure to gas

Guide to Postoperative Respiratory Complications

If your patient's had major surgery, he faces the risk of developing one of the respiratory complications described here. Safeguard your patient by making sure you can quickly recognize a developing problem; then, take appropriate action.

ATELECTASIS

(Incomplete expansion of alveoli or lung segments, which may result in partial or total lung collapse. After surgery, this is usually caused by excessive secretions or a mucus plug.)

Contributing factors
• Administration of gas anesthetics with high oxygen and low nitrogen concentrations
• Prolonged intubation of left or right main stem bronchus, which predisposes lung on opposite side to atelectasis
• Inadequate suctioning during intubation, allowing bronchial secretions to accumulate
• Suppression of cough reflex by sedatives or anesthetics
• Failure to adequately deep breathe and cough following abdominal or thoracic surgery, from incisional pain or a tight-fitting dressing
• Dehydration
• Prolonged immobilization after surgery
• Impaired alveolar function; for example, from chronic obstructive pulmonary disease (COPD)
• Weak respiratory muscles
• Elevated diaphragm; for example, from abdominal gas, bleeding, or tumor

Signs and symptoms
• Dyspnea and cyanosis
• Tachycardia
• Diminished or absent breath sounds on auscultation
• Flatness on percussion
• Decreased chest expansion
• Decreased blood pressure
• Increased temperature
• Restlessness
• Confusion

Nursing interventions
• Encourage patient to deep breathe frequently and to cough.
• Administer prophylactic antibiotics, if ordered.
• Administer humidified air or oxygen, with or without a mucolytic drug, to loosen secretions, as ordered.
• If ordered, use chest percussion (or vibration) along with postural drainage to help clear secretions. To encourage gravitational drainage, position the patient so the affected lung area is elevated above unaffected areas. Perform nasotracheal suctioning, if needed. (This procedure may require a doctor's order, so check your hospital's policy.)

Continued

Guide to Postoperative Respiratory Complications
Continued

ATELECTASIS
Continued

• Prepare the patient for possible deep suctioning by bronchoscopy, a procedure performed by the doctor.
• Administer intermittent positive pressure breathing (IPPB) therapy, if ordered.
• Begin mechanical ventilation, if ordered.

PNEUMONIA

(Lung inflammation with consolidation)
Contributing factors
• Aspiration of foreign material; for example, vomitus
• Infection
• Atelectasis
• Chemical inhalation
• Prolonged immobilization after surgery
• Dehydration
• Failure to adequately deep breathe and cough after abdominal or thoracic surgery
• Suppression of cough reflex by sedatives or anesthetics
• Impaired alveolar function
• Weak respiratory muscles
Signs and symptoms
• Sudden onset of shaking chills
• Fever
• Flushed skin

• Cough with production of pinkish or rust-colored sputum
• Sharp chest pain in lateral lung fields; increased pain on inspiration
• Headache
• Crackles or rhonchi
• Tachypnea
• Decreased breath sounds from affected lung area
Nursing interventions
• Periodically obtain sputum for culture and sensitivity. To prevent spread of infection, dispose of secretions according to your hospital's infection control standards.
• Encourage the patient to avoid dehydration by drinking plenty of fluids.
• Encourage the patient to frequently deep breathe and cough.
• Administer antibiotics, if ordered.
• If ordered, use chest percussion (or vibration) along with postural drainage to help clear secretions.
• Administer humidified air or oxygen, with or without a mucolytic drug, to loosen secretions (as ordered).
• Perform nasotracheal suctioning, if needed. (This procedure may require a doctor's order.)
• Conserve the patient's energy by providing adequate rest; remember, he may become easily exhausted.

Continued

Guide to Postoperative Respiratory Complications
Continued

PULMONARY EMBOLISM

(Obstruction of pulmonary arterial bed by dislodged thrombus)
Contributing factors
• Prolonged immobility
• Thrombophlebitis
• Prolonged bed rest or immobilization
• Chronic pulmonary disease
• Chronic atrial fibrillation
• Surgery, particularly on the legs, pelvis, abdomen, or thorax
• Lower extremity fracture
• Obesity
• Use of oral contraceptives
• Postpartum period
• Advanced age
• Burns
• Cancer
• Polycythemia
• Sickle cell anemia
• Infection
Signs and symptoms
• Dyspnea
• Tachypnea
• Tachycardia
• Anginal or pleuritic chest pain
• Pleuritic (pleural) friction rub
• Productive cough (sputum may be blood-tinged)
• Crackles (rales) or wheezes during auscultation
• Low-grade fever
• Low PaO_2 and $PaCO_2$ values
• Cyanosis
• Syncope

• Neck vein distention
• Hypoxemia
• Restlessness
• Anxiety
• Severe hypotension
• Cardiac dysrhythmias
• Hemoptysis
Nursing interventions
• Administer oxygen by face mask or nasal cannula, as ordered.
• Be prepared to intubate the patient, if necessary.
• Prepare the patient for a chest X-ray and lung scan.
• Connect patient to a cardiac monitor, or obtain frequent EKGs.
• Implement anticoagulant drug therapy, as ordered. *Important:* If the doctor's ordered heparin sodium (Lipo-Hepin), have protamine sulfate on hand to neutralize the heparin sodium, if necessary.
• Obtain blood coagulation studies, and closely monitor them.
• Elevate head of bed to relieve dyspnea.
• Monitor arterial blood gas measurements, as ordered.
• Monitor fluid intake and output. Insert an indwelling (Foley) catheter, if ordered.
• Administer an analgesic, as ordered, to relieve pain and anxiety.
• Conserve the patient's energy by providing adequate rest.

What You Should Know about Epistaxis

Epistaxis (nosebleed) is usually resolved quickly with proper medical attention, but severe epistaxis can be life-threatening. In all cases, assess the cause and type of epistaxis quickly and then provide the necessary care.

What causes epistaxis? Here are some possibilities:
• Upper respiratory tract or sinus infections, which lead to forceful nose blowing
• Habitual nose picking or rubbing
• Low indoor humidity, which dries out the nasal membranes
• Cardiovascular disease
• Head trauma
• Medications that thin the blood, such as aspirin and anticoagulants
• History of bleeding tendencies associated with leukemia and aplastic anemia
• Allergies

In most cases, epistaxis begins in the *anterior* nasal septum. Blood may flow from one or both nasal cavities. When epistaxis originates in the *posterior* nasal septum, the condition's more serious.

Blood may flow from both nasal cavities into the mouth and throat, possibly obstructing the airway.

If your patient has severe epistaxis, control the bleeding before taking his history. If the epistaxis is mild, ask him these questions:
• When did the bleeding begin? Is the blood flowing from one or both nostrils?
• Have you had nosebleeds in the past? How frequently? When was the last time?
• Do you usually have trouble stopping the bleeding?
• Were you hit in the face recently?
• Have you had a cold or sinus problems recently? Have you noticed any sores or tenderness inside your nose?
• Do you have any allergies?
• Have you been treated for hypertension, heart disease, or a blood disorder?
• Have you noticed any other bleeding?
• Have you had oral or nasal surgery recently?
• Are you taking any medications regularly? What? How often?

Nasal Balloon Catheters

To control posterior epistaxis, the doctor may use a nasal balloon catheter instead of posterior nasal packing. These catheters are self-retaining and disposable, and can be either single- or double-cuffed. The single-cuffed catheter (see left illustration below) consists of a cuff that, when inflated, compresses the blood vessels, and a soft, collapsible outside bulb that prevents the catheter from slipping out of place posteriorly.

The double-cuffed catheter (see right illustration) consists of a posterior cuff that, when inflated, secures the catheter in the nasopharynx; an anterior cuff that, when inflated, compresses the blood vessels; and a central airway that helps the patient breathe more comfortably. Each cuff is inflated independently.

Before insertion, the doctor lubricates the catheter with an antibiotic ointment and inserts it through the patient's nostril.

He then inflates the balloon by inserting sterile saline solution into the appropriate valve. (If a double-cuffed catheter is used, the doctor will inflate the posterior cuff first.) He may secure the catheter by taping its anterior tip to the outside of the patient's nose.

To remove the catheter, the doctor deflates the balloon by inserting the hub of a syringe deeply into the valve and withdrawing the solution. He then gently withdraws the catheter from the nostril.

Check the placement of these catheters routinely. With a double-cuffed catheter, you may clean the central airway with a small-gauge suction catheter *to remove clots or secretions.* The doctor may want to deflate the cuff for 10 minutes every 24 hours *to prevent damage to the patient's nasal mucosa.* Expect to find a small amount of discharge around the catheter each day.

Single-cuffed catheter inflated in place

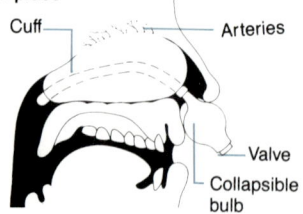

Cuff — Arteries — Valve — Collapsible bulb

Double-cuffed catheter inflated in place

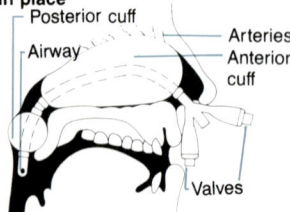

Posterior cuff — Airway — Arteries — Anterior cuff — Valves

Guide to Artificial Airways

ORAL PHARYNGEAL

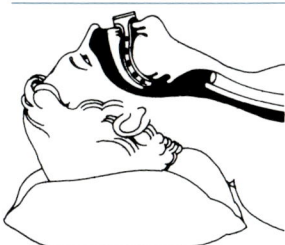

Advantages
- Easy to insert
- Holds tongue away from pharynx
- Inexpensive

Disadvantages
- Easily dislodged
- May stimulate gag reflex

NASAL PHARYNGEAL

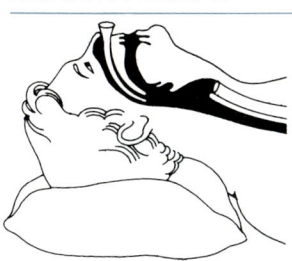

Advantages
- Easy to insert
- Allows for suctioning without displacing the patient's nasal turbinates

Disadvantages
- May cause pressure necrosis
- Kinks and clogs easily, obstructing airway

ORAL ESOPHAGEAL

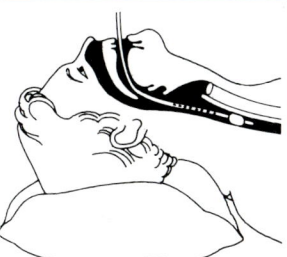

Advantages
- Quick and easy to insert
- Prevents aspiration of stomach contents

Disadvantages
- Expensive
- Presently available in large size only

Continued

MANAGING AIRWAYS

Guide to Artificial Airways
Continued

MANAGING AIRWAYS

ORAL ESOPHAGEAL
Continued

• Can cause pharyngeal trauma during insertion
• Can accidentally enter the trachea, totally obstructing airway
• May cause gastric distention and impaired ventilation if cuff improperly inflated

NASAL ENDOTRACHEAL

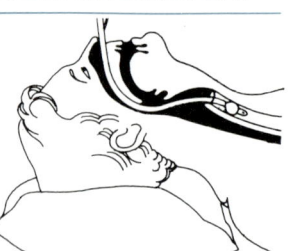

Advantages
• More comfortable than oral endotracheal tube
• Can't be bitten or chewed
• Provides a way to suction
• Can be adapted easily if patient requires continuous ventilation
• Easily anchored in place

Disadvantages
• Kinks and clogs easily, obstructing airway
• Can cause nasal sores, infection, and trauma
• Interferes with cough reflex
• Prevents patient from talking if cuff is inflated
• Tube and cuff can cause tracheal damage

ORAL ENDOTRACHEAL

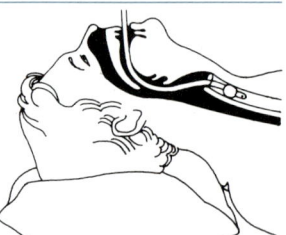

Advantages
• Causes less intubation trauma than nasal endotracheal airway
• Permits use of a larger diameter tube
Disadvantages
• Kinks and clogs easily, obstructing airway

Continued

Guide to Artificial Airways
Continued

ORAL ENDOTRACHEAL
Continued

- Interferes with cough reflex
- Prevents patient from talking if cuff is inflated
- Can be bitten or chewed
- Can cause pressure sores
- Uncomfortable; can stimulate retching, which may lead to gastric distention
- Can cause tracheal damage

TRACHEOSTOMY

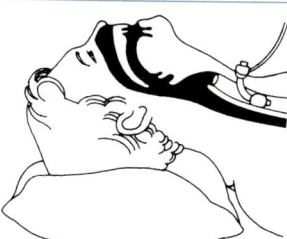

Advantages
- Can be suctioned more easily than an endotracheal tube
- Decreases amount of dead air space in respiratory system
- Permits patient to swallow
- More comfortable for the patient and less likely to become dislodged than the oral or nasal endotracheal tube

Disadvantages
- Requires surgery to insert
- Can cause tracheal damage, especially in children
- Prevents patient from talking if cuff is inflated.

LARYNGECTOMY

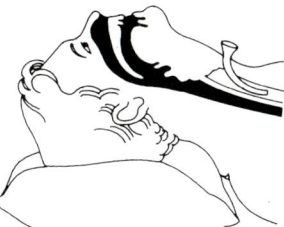

Advantages
- Provides a patent airway
- Eliminates danger of aspiration
- Decreases amount of dead air space in respiratory system

Disadvantages
- Permanent airway
- Deprives patient of normal speech

Artificial Airway Problems

TRACHEOESOPHAGEAL FISTULA

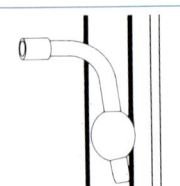

Suspect it when
• You detect an air leak through the stoma or nose and mouth although cuff is up.
• You suction the patient's airway and observe food or liquid in the aspirate.
• The patient belches frequently.
• The patient coughs every time he swallows.
• You get positive results from a methylene blue test.

To intervene
• Don't feed the patient until the extent of the fistula is determined.
• Suction his trachea through the tube only.

To avoid the complication
• Use a low-pressure cuff and the minimal leak technique.
• Exercise meticulous cuff care.

SECRETIONS OBSTRUCT TUBE LUMEN

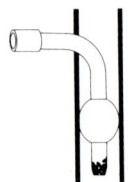

Suspect it when
• You feel an obstruction in the tube when suctioning.

To intervene
• Move suction catheter to one side to pass obstruction.
• Instill saline, hyperinflate the patient's lungs, and suction him with a correct-sized catheter.
• The doctor may want to change the tube, order bronchodilator drugs, or give the patient I.V. therapy.
• Humidify the patient's airway.
• Perform meticulous trach care.
• Perform postural drainage, percussion, and vibration.

To avoid the complication
• Use humidified oxygen to keep secretions thin.

Continued

Artificial Airway Problems
Continued

RUPTURED CUFF

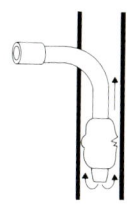

Suspect it when
• You detect a significant air leak through the stoma, nose, or mouth.
• No pressure registers on a manometer check.
• The ventilator shows a decrease in the patient's expired volume.
• The ventilator's low-pressure alarm sounds.
To intervene
• Notify the doctor and prepare to change the tube.
To avoid the complication
• Check the cuff's symmetry by inflating it before insertion.
• Avoid accidentally pulling the cuff into the suction catheter when you're performing nasotracheal suctioning.

HERNIATED CUFF BLOCKING THE END OF THE TUBE

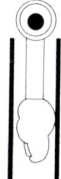

Suspect it when
• You feel an obstruction in the tube when you're suctioning.
• Low-pressure alarm sounds on patient's ventilator.
• Patient experiences moderate difficulty on inhalation. Exhalation may be completely blocked.
To intervene
• Replace the tube immediately. Have a replacement on hand.
To avoid the complication
• Check the cuff for symmetrical inflation *before* you insert the tube.
• Avoid overinflation of the cuff.

Continued

MANAGING AIRWAYS

Artificial Airway Problems
Continued

MANAGING AIRWAYS

CARINA OR WALL OF TRACHEA OBSTRUCTS TUBE LUMEN

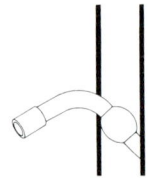

Suspect it when
- You have difficulty forcing air into the tube with a hand ventilator.
- You feel an obstruction in the tube when you're suctioning.
- You note that the patient's blood gas measurement shows a decrease in PaO_2.
- The ventilator's pressure alarm sounds.
- The patient seems anxious and agitated (air hunger).

To intervene
- Deflate cuff and reposition tube.

To avoid the complication
- Make sure you select the proper size tube.
- Tape the tubing securely.
- Tie the trach ties snugly.

UNDERINFLATED CUFF

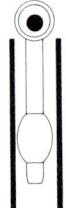

Suspect it when
- You detect a significant air leak through the stoma, nose, or mouth.
- The ventilator shows a decrease in the patient's expired volume.

To intervene
- Inflate the cuff to the proper size. Make sure you use the minimal leak technique.

To avoid the complication
- Follow the manufacturer's recommendations on cuff volume as an initial guide, but then use the minimal leak technique.
- Measure cuff pressure immediately after inflation, and routinely check pressure.

Choosing the Correct Tube Size

Is the doctor about to perform a tracheotomy or intubate your patient? Use the chart on pages 130-131 to help you assemble the correct size tubing. Then, observe the following important guidelines:

● Always examine the patient *before* you consider tubing size. Look for unusual features or conditions that may affect the size of his nasal or oral passage: for example, overdeveloped neck muscles; a relatively small nose; signs of tracheal or epiglottal edema (wheezing or stridor).

● When you know the range of recommended sizes for your particular patient, select the tube with the largest internal diameter. It'll permit better gas flow.

● The patient who'll undergo a tracheotomy may need an adjust-ment in trach tube size once postop edema diminishes. Watch for an enlargement in stoma size, which'll indicate the swelling has gone down. Notify the doctor.

● Don't expect to find cuffs on tracheostomy and endotracheal tubes under size 5 or 5.5 (generally used to intubate children). In a child, cuff pressure is hard to regulate and may cause severe damage.

● If the doctor specifies a Shiley tracheostomy tube, remember you can only get it in even sizes: 4, 6, 8, or 10.

● Suppose you know the internal diameter of an endotracheal tube and want the French size. To get it, multiply the diameter by 4.

Nursing Tip

When removing a patient's oral endotracheal tube, have him take deep breaths as tube is removed to open vocal cords and prevent trauma. To remove the tube, deflate the cuff, hold a washcloth over the patient's chest, and pull the tube out in a smooth, slightly downward motion. Take care not to damage the patient's trachea. Offer the patient an emesis basin if he needs it. Removing the tube may have stimulated his gag reflex.

Immediately after you remove the tube, give the patient humidified oxygen by face mask at prescribed flow. Cough and deep-breathe him. Let him expectorate. Then give him proper mouth care, including a mouthwash. Remove tape marks from the patient's cheeks.

Guide to Endotracheal and Tracheostomy Tube Sizes

Use the chart below to help you assemble the correct tube size for a tracheostomy or intubation. Remember—always examine the patient *before* you consider tubing size.

AGE OF PATIENT	ENDOTRACHEAL TUBE (I.D.)	(FR)
Newborn	3.0 mm	12
6 months	3.5 mm	14
18 months	4.0 mm	16
3 years	4.5 mm	18
5 years	5.0 mm	20
6 years	5.5 mm	22
8 years	6.0 mm	24
12 years	6.5 mm	26
16 years	7.0 mm	28
Adult (female)	7.0 to 8.5 mm	32 to 34
Adult (male)	8.5 to 10.0 mm	34 to 40

MANAGING AIRWAYS

Look for unusual features or conditions that may affect the size of his nasal or oral passage: for example, overdeveloped neck muscles; a relatively small nose; signs of tracheal or epiglottal edema (wheezing or stridor).

TRACH (I.D.)	SIZE	SUCTION CATHETER (FR)
4 to 5 mm	00.0	6
5.5 mm	1.0	8
6.0 mm	1.2	8
6 to 7 mm	2.3	8
7.0 mm	3.0	10
7.0 mm	3.0	10
8.0 mm	4.0	10
9.0 mm	5.0	10
9.0 mm	6.0	10
9 to 11 mm	6 to 10	12 to 14
9 to 11 mm	6 to 10	14 to 18

Using a Nasal Pharyngeal Airway

Suppose your patient needs a nasal pharyngeal airway. Could you insert it correctly? How can you tell if the tube's in the right position? Do you know how to remove it with the least discomfort for your patient? If you're not sure, read the following:

Inserting the tube
Determine the correct tube length for your patient. To do this, measure from the tip of his nose to his earlobe. Mark the distance on the tube. For a snug fit, use a tube with an outside diameter slightly larger than the patient's nostril.

Next, lubricate the tube with water or a soluble jelly. Reassure your patient and explain what you're going to do. Then, push up the tip of his nose and insert the tube into his nostril up to the mark you've made.

If patient gags
If the patient with a nasal pharyngeal airway coughs or gags, it may indicate that the tube is too long. If so, remove the airway and insert a shorter one.

Tube care
Once every 8 hours, remove the airway *to check nasal mucous membranes for irritation or ulceration.* Clean the airway by placing

it in a basin and rinsing it with hydrogen peroxide and then with water. If secretions remain, use a pipe cleaner to remove them. Reinsert the clean airway into the other nostril, if it's patent, *to avoid skin breakdown.*

Checking the tube's position
Ask the patient to exhale with mouth closed. You'll know the tube's in place if you feel air coming through it. Check the tube's position visually, too. Hold the patient's mouth open with a tongue blade, and look for the tube's tip just behind the uvula.

Administering oxygen
To increase oxygen availability during respiration, insert a nasal catheter through the airway or place a nasal cannula just under the nose.

Removing the tube
First, tell the patient what you're going to do. Then suction the tube to remove collected secretions. When you've completed that, withdraw the tube in one smooth motion. If it's stuck, *don't* use force. Instead, apply lubricant around tube and nostril, and gently rotate the tube until it's free. Document what you've done in your nurses' notes.

Tracheotomy or Tracheostomy: What's the Difference?

Do these terms confuse you? Study the definitions below to learn how they differ.
Tracheotomy: an opening made surgically to alleviate respiratory distress.
Tracheostomy: the surgical incision created by the tracheotomy.

Tracheotomy Indications

When does your patient need a tracheotomy? Usually, the doctor only performs a tracheotomy in the operating room. But in an emergency, when every second counts, he may perform a tracheotomy at the patient's bedside
• when other methods fail to relieve an obstructed airway
• when acute laryngeal edema closes or threatens to close the patient's airway
• when he needs long-term airway management or prolonged mechanical ventilation
• when he can't tolerate an endotracheal tube; for example, in cases of severe mouth or facial injuries
• when physiologic dead air space lessens the patient's FIO_2.

Chances are, the doctor will avoid a tracheotomy in these situations:
• when infection risk is great; for example, when the patient has profound leukopenia
• when the patient needs only short-term airway management or mechanical ventilation
• when the patient has a serious bleeding disorder; for example, disseminated intravascular coagulation (DIC).

How to Prepare Your Patient for a Bedside Tracheotomy

As you know, the doctor usually performs a tracheotomy under strict surgical asepsis. However, he may have to do one at the patient's bedside. If he does, here's how to help.

First, assemble the following equipment and have it ready: trach tray, sterile gloves, Betadine, sterile water, size 3-0 and 4-0 silk sutures, and a local anesthetic. In addition to this, gather the equipment you need for suctioning during or after the procedure; suction catheters, gloves, and sterile saline.

Be sure to check the charts on pages 130-131 as a guideline for choosing the correct size tracheostomy tube.

Make sure the patient or an appropriate person has signed the proper surgical consent form, and get it witnessed. Always check the hospital's policy regarding consent forms *before* you get them signed.

When you've accomplished all this, prepare the patient for the procedure by explaining what to expect. Position him flat on his back. Place a small rolled towel under his shoulder blades to hyperextend his neck and properly align his mouth and trachea.

Remove the bed's headboard, so you can quickly get behind the patient's head to mechanically ventilate him, if necessary.

Make sure the procedure area is well lighted.

In the illustration at right, you'll see where the doctor makes the incision for a tracheotomy. Note how its position differs from that of the cricoid stab shown on page 136.

In a tracheotomy, the doctor must first split the patient's thyroid gland and hold it back with retractors. Then he can make the incision in the trachea below the cricoid cartilage.

Continued

How to Prepare Your Patient for a Bedside Tracheotomy
Continued

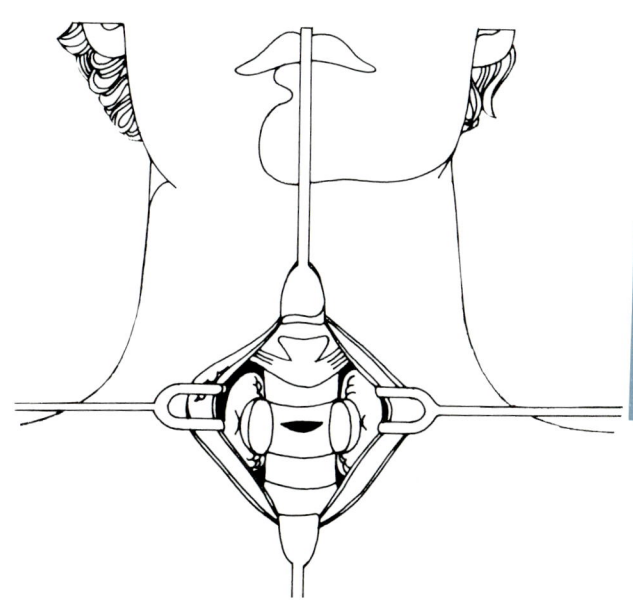

How to Do a Cricoid Stab

Suppose you're the only health-care professional at an accident scene, and you know the victim needs an emergency tracheotomy. This illustration will show you where to do a cricoid stab. Simply cut or stab the victim's cricothyroid membrane between the thyroid cartilage and the cricoid ring. Then, insert something hollow to keep the airway open.

Important: Obviously, you'd never attempt such a procedure in the hospital. You'd do it only in an extreme emergency situation like the one described here.

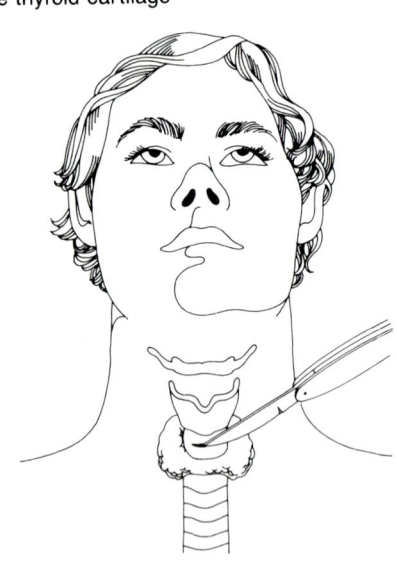

Caring for a Tracheostomy

• Treat the tracheostomy site as a surgical wound. Use sterile technique, wear gloves, and wash your hands before and after suctioning.

• Change dressing (sterile, precut gauze) every 8 hours.

• Suction as needed but only during withdrawal of the catheter and only 5 to 10 seconds at a time.

• Allow the patient to breathe, or ventilate him with a ventilator, after each passage of the catheter.

• Ventilate the patient with 100% oxygen (with an Ambu bag, if necessary) before, during, and after each suctioning.

• Avoid too-vigorous suctioning, which could cause severe tracheal injury.

• Change the sterile humidifier and nebulizer every 24 hours; change sterile water and tubing every 8 hours.

• Discard water condensed in tubing as necessary.

• Routinely culture tracheal aspirate at least every 3 days. Check and record color change, consistency, and amount of secretions.

• Inspect the site frequently for bleeding, hematoma formation, and possible dissection of air through the tissue of the neck.

• When the patient is to begin oral feeding, offer water first to make sure he can swallow without aspirating.

• Deflate the cuff only if a significant change occurs in the airway pressure.

Nursing Tip

To make your trach patient more comfortable, incorporate these tips in his daily care plan.

• *Help him communicate.* The trach patient who's dependent on a ventilator will be frustrated by his inability to communicate. Be understanding and supportive when he's irritable. Help him find new ways to express himself by giving him a writing tablet, picture cards, magic slate, or chalkboard. Try to interpret his body language.

• *Help him cough up secretions.* To do this, instruct him to inhale deeply and cough. If his tracheostomy's covered when he coughs, the secretions will collect in his nose and mouth. If the tracheostomy isn't covered, they'll exit through his trach tube. Have tissues ready. Also, remind the patient to cover both his nose *and* his tracheostomy when he sneezes.

Special Considerations for Tracheostomy Care

For immediate use in an emergency, always have ready the following: all equipment and supplies for suctioning, *since the patient may need his airway cleared at any time;* the sterile obturator originally used to insert the patient's tracheostomy tube, *for quick reinsertion if the tube is expelled;* an additional sterile tracheostomy tube (with obturator) of the size currently being used, *to replace a contaminated or expelled tube;* and a spare sterile inner cannula, *to replace a contaminated or expelled inner cannula.* Additional emergency equipment (optional): sterile tracheostomy tube (with obturator) one size smaller than that currently being used, *to replace an expelled tube when the trachea immediately begins to close, making difficult the insertion of a tube of the original size;* a sterile tracheal dilator or sterile hemostat, *to maintain an open airway before insertion of a new tracheostomy tube.*

Refrain from changing tracheostomy ties unnecessarily during the immediate postoperative period before the stoma track is well formed (usually 4 days) *to avoid accidental dislodgement and expulsion of the tube.* Unless secretions or drainage are a problem, ties can be changed once a day.

Refrain from changing a single-cannula tracheostomy tube or the outer cannula of a double-cannula tube. Because of the risk of tracheal complications, the doctor usually changes the cannula, with the frequency of change depending on the patient's condition (once a week or every other week is usual). For patients going home with a metal tracheostomy tube, the usual procedure is to teach the patient to change the tube and clean it daily.

If the patient's neck or stoma is excoriated or infected, apply a water-soluble topical lubricant or antibiotic cream as ordered. Remember not to use a powder or an oil-based substance on or around a stoma *because aspiration can cause infection and abscess.*

Guide to Tracheostomy Tubes

What makes the doctor choose one type of tracheostomy tube over another in a particular situation? This chart will give you some answers.

PLASTIC, CUFFED (HIGH-PRESSURE)

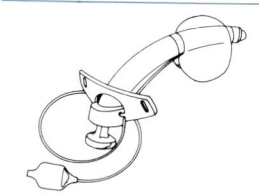

Advantages
• Disposable
• Cuff bonded to tube; won't detach accidentally inside trachea

Disadvantages
• More likely to cause tracheal damage or tissue necrosis than low-pressure cuff

PLASTIC, DOUBLE-CUFFED (HIGH-PRESSURE)

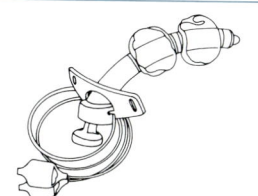

Advantages
➲ Reduces risk of tissue necrosis because cuffs can be inflated alternately

Disadvantages
• May be difficult to insert
• Tracheal damage, if it occurs, will cover a larger area
• Will reduce risk of tissue necrosis *only* when you rigidly adhere to alternate inflation schedule

PLASTIC, CUFFED (LOW-PRESSURE)

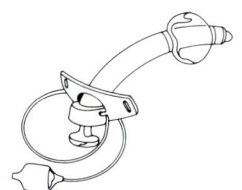

Advantages
• Disposable
• Cuff bonded to tube; won't detach accidentally inside trachea   *Continued*

Guide to Tracheostomy Tubes
Continued

PLASTIC, CUFFED (LOW-
PRESSURE)
Continued

• Cuff pressure low and evenly
distributed against trachea
wall; no need to deflate periodically to reduce pressure
• Decreases risk of tracheal
damage
Disadvantages
• More costly

METAL, CUFFED (HIGH- OR
LOW-PRESSURE)

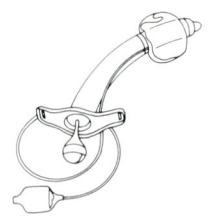

Advantages
• Available in small sizes for
infants
• Inner cannula can be removed for easy cleaning or
sterilization
• Removable cuff makes it
easy to sterilize tube

Disadvantages
• Cuff tears easily if you try
to remove it
• Cuff can slip off easily
• Inner cannula easily dis-
lodged
• Adapter needed with some
types to ventilate patient

PLASTIC OR METAL, UN-
CUFFED

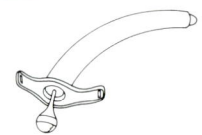

Advantages
• Reduces risk of tracheal
damage to minimum
• Recommended for children
because they don't require
cuff
• Permits free flow of air
around tube and through larynx
Disadvantages
• In adults, lack of cuff increases risk of aspiration and
prevents mechanical ventilation.

Tracheostomy Attachments: How They Work

ONE-WAY TRACH VALVE BOX

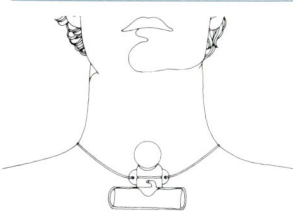

What it does: enables the tracheostomy patient to speak.

How it works
• The valve box fits into the trach tube opening. When the patient inhales, the one-way valve lets air through the trach tube into his lungs. When he exhales, the force of his breath closes the valve. This diverts air through the larynx and enables him to speak.

Nursing tip
• Don't use a one-way valve on a patient who has an inflated cuff or tight-fitting tube. Why? Such a patient can't exhale.

ARTIFICIAL NOSE

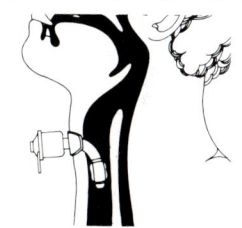

What it does: provides humidification.

How it works
• The artificial nose fits directly onto the tracheostomy tube. As the patient exhales, the artificial nose traps moisture. Then, as he inhales, the moisture evaporates again.

Nursing tip
• The artificial nose is best for ambulatory patients who don't need oxygen therapy.

Continued

MANAGING AIRWAYS

Tracheostomy Attachments: How They Work
Continued

TRACHEOSTOMY BUTTON

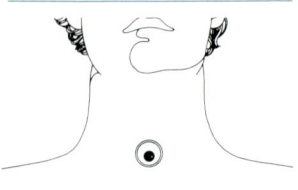

What it does: helps wean the patient from tracheostomy.

How it works
● A tracheostomy button consists of a short outer tube that fits into the stoma and reaches the trachea, and a solid cannula that completely closes the tube.

Nursing tip
● To give nebulizer treatments, insert an adapter cannula through the outer cannula into the patient's trachea.

TRACHEOSTOMY PLUG

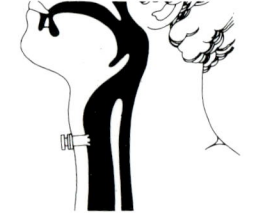

What it does: helps wean the patient from tracheostomy.

How it works
● A tracheostomy plug fits into the outer cannula of most small-diameter tracheostomy tubes. To wean the patient, gradually decrease the trach tube diameter. Then plug his trach tube completely, making it necessary for the patient to breathe normally.

Nursing tip
● Deflate the cuff as you begin weaning.

Problems with Tracheostomies

TUBE OUT OF PLACE

How to recognize it
Trach tube doesn't enter trachea properly during insertion. Instead, it lodges in the surrounding tissues, making it difficult and painful for patient to breathe. This problem occurs most commonly in patients with overdeveloped neck muscles.

How to remedy it
• If you can't find a long enough trach tube to substitute for the first one, the doctor can insert an endotracheal tube into the stoma. After it's inserted properly, make sure you leave at least 2″ outside stoma for adapter.

How to prevent it
• If the patient has overdeveloped neck muscles, anticipate a problem. Use a trach tube that's both longer and larger.
• If the patient's on a ventilator, prevent the ventilator tubing from pulling on his trach tube and dislodging it. Support ventilator tubing with a rolled towel or washcloth.

SUBCUTANEOUS EMPHYSEMA

How to recognize it
Air escapes from trachea into surrounding soft tissues. This prob-
lem occurs most commonly in patients who are being mechanically ventilated. Inspect for crepitus in the neck tissues. Listen for air escaping around trach tube cuff.

How to remedy it
• Check to make sure the cuff's properly inflated. The doctor may want to insert a larger tracheostomy tube. Document extent of crepitus.

How to prevent it
• Always use correct size trach tube. (To determine this, see the chart on pages 130-131.)

PNEUMOTHORAX

How to recognize it
There'll be decreased or no breath sounds on the affected side. In some cases, the patient will also have subcutaneous emphysema, tachypnea, and pain on the affected side.

How to remedy it
• In some cases, the doctor will choose to insert a chest tube or flutter valve. Or he may let a small pneumothorax resolve itself.

How to prevent it
• Watch for subcutaneous emphysema, which may indicate impending pneumothorax. Notify doctor.

Continued

MANAGING AIRWAYS

Problems with Tracheostomies
Continued

MANAGING AIRWAYS

BLEEDING AROUND INSERTION SITE

How to recognize it
Excessive postop bleeding may occur. In most cases, the patient will have only slight bleeding after a properly performed tracheotomy, unless he has a bleeding disorder or the trach tube becomes dislodged.

How to remedy it
● Keep the trach cuff inflated to prevent edema and keep patient from aspirating blood.
● Don't administer heated humidity while the patient is bleeding.
● Document the rate and amount of bleeding by noting the number of saturated gauze pads.
● Assist the doctor if he wants to apply Gelfoam to a small bleeder or ligate it.
● Ask the doctor if he wants to order blood coagulation studies from the laboratory.

How to prevent it
● Don't pull on the trach tube.
● Instruct the patient not to pull or tug on the trach tube, as it can irritate the surrounding tissue and cause bleeding.
● If trach dressing's coagulated to the fresh trach site, wet it with hydrogen peroxide. Never pull it off abruptly.

INFECTION AT TRACHEOSTOMY SITE

How to recognize it
Patient will have purulent, foul-smelling drainage coming from tracheostomy. He may also have a slightly elevated temperature, malaise, increased WBC count, local pain or discomfort.

How to remedy it
● Document your findings and notify the doctor immediately. He'll want to order culture and sensitivity tests and possibly prescribe a systemic antibiotic.
● Inflate the trach cuff so the patient doesn't aspirate any drainage.
● Suction patient frequently, maintaining sterile technique.
● Avoid cross-contamination.
● Change trach dressing whenever soiled.
● Watch for improvement in drainage and document your findings.

How to prevent it
● Always use strict sterile technique for trach care.
● Thoroughly clean ventilator and oxygen tubing.
● Change all tubing and nebulizer or humidifier jar daily.
● Collect sputum and wound drainage specimens for culture studies.

How to Reinsert a Trach Tube in an Emergency

Anytime you're caring for a patient with a trach tube, you risk that he'll cough up the tube and you'll have to reinsert it. Prepare for this emergency by having a sterile trach tube at the bedside. However, if you don't have one, use the dislodged tube and proceed as follows:

• Reassure the patient.

• Remove the inner cannula from the dislodged trach tube after you deflate the cuff.

• Take the obturator, which is usually on the bedside table or taped to the head of the bed, and insert it into the trach's outer cannula.

• Reinsert the trach tube (with the obturator) into the patient's stoma.

• Hold the trach plate in place while you remove the obturator and insert the inner cannula into the trach tube.

• Turn the inner cannula clockwise until it locks in place. (Chances are, your patient will cough or gag while you're doing this, so be sure to hold onto the trach plate securely to prevent the same emergency from recurring.)

• Remove the needle from a syringe, and insert the tip of the syringe into the tube's pillow port.

• Inflate the cuff and secure the trach ties.

• Put the bib around the trach plate.

• Auscultate his lungs to make sure he's getting air.

• Reassure your patient that he will be able to breathe as before.

• Tell him that you've firmly secured his trach tube.

• Take time to stay with him till he's relaxed.

• Document the entire episode on the patient's chart.

Esophageal Airway Insertion

In a respiratory crisis occurring outside the hospital, such specially trained personnel as emergency medical technicians may have to insert an esophageal gastric tube airway (EGTA) or an esophageal obturator airway (EOA) in the patient.

The **esophageal obturator airway** consists of an adjustable, inflatable, transparent face mask with a single port, attached by a snap lock to a blind esophageal tube.

When properly inflated, the transparent mask prevents air from escaping through the nose and mouth. (See top illustration on opposite page.)

The esophageal tube has 16 holes at its proximal end through which air or oxygen, blown into the port of the mask, is transferred to the trachea.

The tube's distal end is closed and circled by an inflatable cuff. When the cuff is inflated, it occludes the esophagus, preventing air from entering the stomach and acting as a barrier against vomitus and involuntary aspiration.

This cuff rests in the esophagus just below the tracheal bifurcation to prevent pressure on the noncartilaginous back of the tracheal wall.

The **esophageal gastric tube airway** consists of an inflatable face mask and an esophageal tube. The transparent face mask has two ports: a lower port for insertion of a nasogastric tube and an upper port for ventilation. The inside of the mask is soft and pliable; it molds to the patient's face and makes a tight seal, preventing air loss.

A gastric (Levin) tube can be used to suction stomach contents before extubation. It's inserted through the mask's lower port into the esophageal tube, then through a small hole in the end of the tube.

The distal end of the tube has an inflatable cuff like that of the EOA.

During ventilation, air is blown into the upper port in the mask and, with the esophagus blocked, enters the trachea and lungs. (See bottom illustration.)

Continued

Esophageal Airway Insertion
Continued

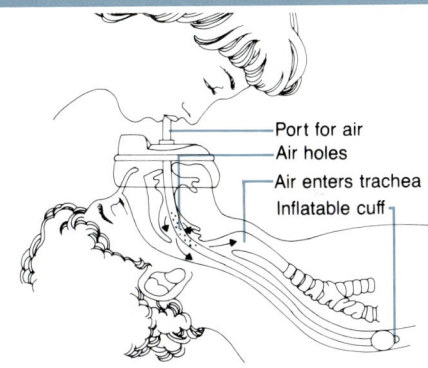

Port for air
Air holes
Air enters trachea
Inflatable cuff

Esophageal obturator airway

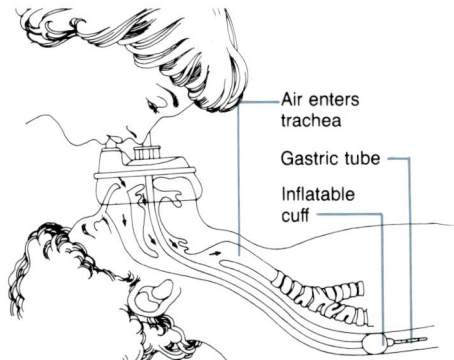

Air enters trachea
Gastric tube
Inflatable cuff

Esophageal gastric tube airway

Does Your Patient Need Suctioning?

Prepare to suction your patient any time he's unable to cough up secretions that obstruct his airway. This can happen when:
• he has a neuromuscular disorder that keeps him from coughing; for example, Guillain-Barré syndrome.
• he has unusually heavy or thick secretions; for example, from pulmonary edema or cystic fibrosis.
• he's lost his cough reflex from head injury, anesthesia, or drug overdose.
• his airway is obstructed by an endotracheal tube or his jaws are wired shut after reconstructive surgery.

Watch for these danger signs that indicate your patient may require regular suctioning:
• dyspnea
• tachycardia
• audible crackles, diminished breath sounds
• restlessness, agitation
• rhonchi, and gurgling over large airways.

Also, listen for the ventilator's pressure alarm to go off. This may indicate that the patient's airway is partially obstructed and he needs suctioning. Use caution suctioning your patient if he's had recent surgery on his nose, throat, esophagus, or trachea.

Suction cautiously through his nasopharynx if he has a blood dyscrasia or is on anticoagulants. Never suction if he shows signs of a cerebrospinal fluid leak, or active bleeding from his nasopharynx. *Nursing tip:* To detect a cerebrospinal fluid leak, watch for a halo around stains caused by nasal secretions.

How well is your patient tolerating the procedure? Watch for these signs of complications:
• bloody aspirant, indicating possible nasal or tracheal damage
• cardiac dysrhythmias, particularly bradycardia or atrioventricular (AV) heart block
• cyanosis, indicating hypoxemia
• laryngospasm.

Do your best to prevent dysrhythmias, hypoxemia, or bronchospasms from occurring by giving your patient an increased amount of oxygen before you begin suctioning. *Important:* In cases of laryngospasm, you may find it hard to remove the suction catheter. Don't try. Instead, disconnect the tube connecting the suction catheter to the suction equipment, and let the catheter act as an artificial airway.

After any suctioning, auscultate the patient's lungs to make sure the suctioning was effective. Remember to chart your findings.

Suctioning Problems: How to Solve and Avoid Them

Problem:
You attempt to suction a patient and discover the equipment doesn't suction.

Here's what to do
• Make sure unit is plugged in (if it's electric).
• Make sure the unit is securely attached to wall socket.
• Check fit on vacuum bottle lid.
• Make sure tubing and catheter connections aren't loose.
• Check switch to make sure it's on.
• Make sure catheter isn't kinked.
To avoid problem next time
• Check equipment carefully at the beginning of each shift.
• Draw some sterile water or saline solution through the suction catheter to check it before you insert the catheter into the patient.

Problem:
Patient goes into bronchospasm while you're suctioning him, and you're unable to remove catheter with gentle tugging.

Here's what to do
• Don't use force to remove it.
• Disconnect catheter from the connecting tubing, and let it act as an airway.
• If bronchospasm doesn't subside immediately, give the patient oxygen by placing oxygen tube to

catheter end and increasing prescribed liter flow.
• When bronchospasm does subside, quickly remove catheter, and give patient prescribed amount of oxygen. Reassure him.
To avoid problem next time
• Suction patient only when necessary. If possible, get him to cough up secretions.
• Suction gently.
• If patient's having difficulty, remove catheter before he has bronchospasm and give oxygen.

Problem:
Your patient sounds congested, but you're unable to suction any secretions from his endotracheal tube or trach tube. Or, the secretions you *do* suction are extremely dry or viscous.

Here's what to do
• Using a syringe (with the needle removed), instill 2 to 3 ml saline solution into the endotracheal tube or trach tube.
• Hyperinflate the patient's lungs with a hand-held ventilator.
• Proceed with suctioning.
• Repeat procedure again later, if necessary, but only after you've given patient a chance to rest.
To avoid problem next time
• Keep patient well hydrated.
• Administer humidification ther-
Continued

MANAGING AIRWAYS

Suctioning Problems: How to Solve and Avoid Them
Continued

apy and aerosol treatments, as ordered. Or request an order from the doctor.
• Don't give milk or milk products to patient, because they can thicken and increase sputum.

Problem:
You're suctioning the mouth of an aphasic stroke patient and find that he won't cooperate with you.

Here's what to do
• Try to calm him by speaking calmly and soothingly.
• Ask another nurse to keep patient's mouth open with a padded tongue blade. This will keep him from biting down on the catheter.
To avoid problem next time
• Regularly turn the patient from side to side so secretions will drain from his mouth naturally.
• Encourage him to cough up secretions by demonstrating what you want him to do.

Problem:
You're suctioning a patient through his nose and suddenly observe that his heart rate's dropped to 40.

Here's what to do
• Stop suctioning immediately.
• Remove catheter and give oxygen.

• Monitor and document vital signs.
• Notify doctor, if necessary.
To avoid problem next time
• Avoid nasal suctioning unless other methods of removing secretions fail.
• Closely observe patient's heart rate throughout entire procedure.

Problem:
You begin suctioning your patient and notice pink-tinged mucus.

Here's what to do
• Check for signs of pulmonary edema.
• Find out if he's been taking Isuprel, which can cause pink-tinged mucus.
• Ask if he's just eaten red gelatin.
To avoid problem next time
• Keep your patient well hydrated so his mucosa won't get dry and be prone to injury.
• Make sure catheter is correct size. Try a smaller size to minimize trauma.
• Review the technique you're using to make sure it's correct.

Low- and High-Flow
Oxygen and Humidification Delivery Systems

NASAL CANNULA

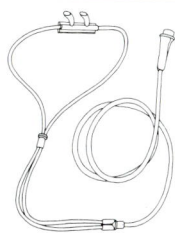

(Low-flow system)
Benefits
- Safe and simple
- Comfortable; easily tolerated
- Nasal prongs can be shaped to fit facial contour
- Effective for delivering low oxygen concentrations
- Allows freedom of movement; doesn't interfere with eating or talking
- Inexpensive; disposable
- Can provide continuous, positive airway pressure for infants and children.

Problems to expect
- Can't be used when patient has complete nasal obstructions; for example, mucosal edema or polyps
- May cause headaches or dry mucous membranes if flow rate exceeds 6 liters/minute
- Can dislodge easily
- Strap may pinch chin if adjusted too tightly
- Patient must be alert and cooperative to help keep cannula in place.

To avoid complications
- Remove and clean cannula every 8 hours with a wet cloth. Give good mouth and nose care.
- If patient's restless, tape cannula in place.
- Check for pressure areas under nose and over ears. Apply gauze padding, if necessary.
- Moisten lips and nose with water-soluble jelly, but take care not to occlude cannula.

Continued

GIVING OXYGEN

Low- and High-Flow
Oxygen and Humidification Delivery Systems
Continued

SIMPLE FACE MASK (Low-flow system)

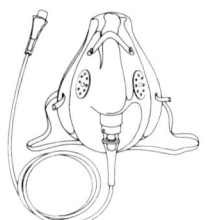

Benefits
• Effectively delivers high oxygen concentrations
• Humidification can be increased by using large-bore tubing and aerosol mask
• Doesn't dry mucous membranes of nose and mouth.
Problems to expect
• Hot and confining; may irritate skin
• Tight seal, necessary for higher oxygen concentration, may cause discomfort
• Interferes with eating and talking
• Can't deliver less than 40% oxygen
• Impractical for long-term therapy.
To avoid complications
• Don't use on patient with COPD.
• Place pads between mask and bony facial parts.
• Periodically massage face with fingertips.
• Wash and dry face every 2 hours.
• For adequate flush, maintain flow rate of 5 liters/minute.
• Don't adjust strap too tightly.
• Remove and clean mask every 8 hours with a wet cloth.

FACE TENT

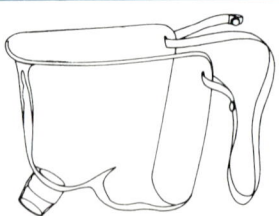

(Humidification system)

Continued

Low- and High-Flow
Oxygen and Humidification Delivery Systems
Continued

FACE TENT
Continued

Benefits
• Provides high humidity
• Functions as a high-flow system when attached to a venturi nebulizer
• Substitutes for face mask if patient can't tolerate having his nose covered; for example, if his nose is broken
• Doesn't dry mucous membranes.

Problems to expect
• Hot and confining; may irritate skin
• Interferes with eating and talking
• Doesn't deliver precise oxygen concentrations without venturi attachment; patient can rebreathe CO_2 unless venturi system is used.
• Impractical for long-term therapy.

To avoid complications
• Same as for simple face mask.
• Watch for signs of oxygen toxicity, especially when a venturi attachment is not used.

PARTIAL REBREATHING
MASK
(Low-flow system)

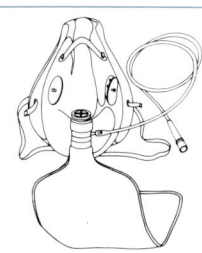

Benefits
• Oxygen reservoir bag lets patient rebreathe his exhaled air, which is high in oxygen content; this increases his fraction inspired oxygen concentration (FIO_2)
• Safety valve allows room air to be inhaled if oxygen source fails
• Effectively delivers higher oxygen concentrations (35% to 60%)
• Easily humidifies oxygen
• Doesn't dry mucous membranes
• By inserting a rubber flange over the reservoir bag, you

Continued

Low- and High-Flow
Oxygen and Humidification Delivery Systems
Continued

PARTIAL REBREATHING
MASK *Continued*

can convert most types to
nonrebreather masks.

Problems to expect
- Tight seal
- Interferes with eating
- Hot and confining; may irritate skin

To avoid complications
- Never let bag totally deflate during inhalation.
- Avoid twisting bag.
- Keep mask snug to prevent inhalation of room air.
- To initially fill bag, apply mask as patient exhales.

NONREBREATHING MASK

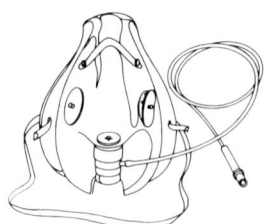

(Low-flow system)
Benefits
- Delivers the highest possible oxygen concentration (60% to 90%) short of intubation and mechanical ventilation
- Effective for short-term therapy
- Doesn't dry mucous membranes
- Can be converted to a partial rebreathing mask, if necessary.

Problems to expect
- Requires a tight seal, which may be difficult to maintain; may cause discomfort
- May irritate skin
- Impractical for long-term therapy.

To avoid complications
- Never let bag totally deflate.
- Avoid twisting bag.
- Keep mask snug to prevent inhalation of room air.
- Make sure that all rubber flaps remain in place.
- Watch patient closely for signs of oxygen toxicity.

Continued

GIVING OXYGEN

Low- and High-Flow
Oxygen and Humidification Delivery Systems
Continued

TRACH COLLAR OR MASK

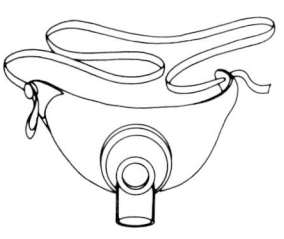

(Humidification system)
Benefits
- Provides high humidity
- Swivel adapter allows tubing to attach on either side
- Frontal port permits suctioning
- Elastic ties allow you to pull mask from tracheostomy without removing it.

Problems to expect
- If condensation's allowed to collect, it can drain into tracheostomy.
- If secretions collect in the collar, stoma can become infected.
- Heated aerosol may cause bleeding if used on fresh trach.

- Intake of room air through the port lowers oxygen concentration.

To avoid complications
- Empty condensation buildup at least once every 2 hours.
- Remove and clean mask every 4 hours with *water*.
- Don't cover exhalation port.
- Make sure nebulizer delivers constant mist.

T-TUBE

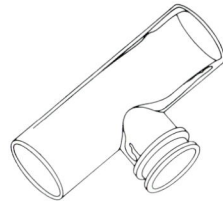

(Humidification system)
Benefits
- Offers high humidity when connected to a nebulizer
- Allows greater patient mobility

Continued

GIVING OXYGEN

Low- and High-Flow
Oxygen and Humidification Delivery Systems
Continued

T-TUBE
Continued

- Can be used for trach or endotrach
- Functions as a high-flow system when attached to a venturi system.

Problems to expect
- May stick to tracheostomy (from humidity or secretions)
- Condensation can collect in tube and drain into tracheostomy.

To avoid complications
- If tube sticks to tracheostomy, gently twist off. Then, clean tube with hydrogen peroxide, rinse with water, and replace.
- Empty condensation buildup at least once every 2 hours.
- Keep chimney extension in place. If you don't, the FIO_2 will drop drastically.
- Make sure humidifier or nebulizer has enough water to create mist.
- Watch for signs of oxygen toxicity, especially if used as a low-flow system.

OXYGEN HOOD

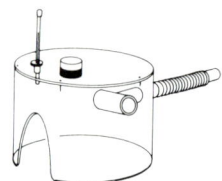

(Humidification system)

Benefits
- Enclosed and compact
- Gives better oxygen concentration than isolette can by itself; lets you care for infant's lower torso
- Functions as a high-flow system when connected to a venturi delivery system
- Offers high humidity when connected to a nebulizer

Problems to expect
- Can irritate skin
- Can't feed infant while he's inside hood
- Active infant can move hood.

To avoid complications
- Pad hood with towel or foam rubber.

Continued

GIVING OXYGEN

Low- and High-Flow
Oxygen and Humidification Delivery Systems
Continued

OXYGEN HOOD
Continued

- Keep bedding around head dry.
- Empty condensation buildup from tubing every 2 hours.
- When using heated nebulizer, check hood temperature every 4 hours so it stays between 94° F. (34.4° C.) and 96° F. (35.6° C.).

ISOLETTE (STANDARD)

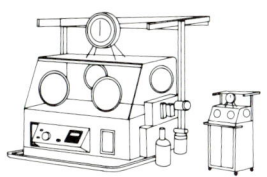

(Low- or high-flow system)
Benefits
- Provides controlled temperature and humidity
- Isolates infants with contagious diseases
- Can be used as a high-flow oxygen system when used

with an oxygen hood.
Problems to expect
- When used without oxygen hood, isolette can deliver only 40% or 100% oxygen. Also, oxygen concentration can fluctuate.
To avoid complications
- If 100% oxygen concentration is desired, keep port flaps closed tightly.
- If oxygen hood isn't used, check oxygen concentration every 4 hours.

CROUPETTE

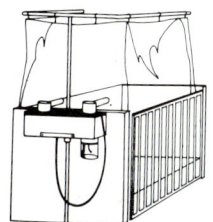

(Low-flow system)
Benefits
- Usually used for children
- Delivers high humidity and aerosolized therapy
Continued

Low- and High-Flow
Oxygen and Humidification Delivery Systems
Continued

GIVING OXYGEN

CROUPETTE
Continued

- Allows child to move freely
- Disposable canopy.

Problems to expect
- If you must open tent, it'll take 15 to 20 minutes to restore oxygen concentration
- Water or ice reservoir must be filled every 6 to 8 hours
- High humidity promotes bacterial growth
- Isolates patient.

To avoid complications
- Check temperature and oxygen concentration every 4 hours.
- Use rubber sheet on bed, to prevent oxygen from escaping through mattress.
- Use bath blanket over bottom sheet to absorb excess moisture; change linen and gown every 2 hours.
- Give care via tent opening when you can. When giving bath or changing linen, tuck tent under pillow to conserve oxygen.

OXYGEN TENT

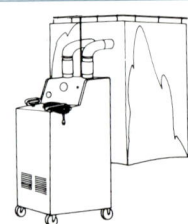

(Low-flow system)

Benefits
- Provides high humidity; temperature can be evenly controlled.

Problems to expect
- If you must open tent, it'll take 15 or 20 minutes to restore oxygen concentration
- High humidity promotes bacterial growth
- Empty tubing at least once every 4 hours
- Isolates patient.

To avoid complications
- Use rubber sheet on bed, to prevent oxygen from escaping through mattress.
- Maintain oxygen flow at 10 to 15 liters/minute for adequate flush.

Continued

Low- and High-Flow
Oxygen and Humidification Delivery Systems
Continued

OXYGEN TENT
Continued

• Check temperature and oxygen concentration every 4 hours; check for leaks in tent.
• Keep patient warm and dry. Give patient care through tent opening whenever possible. When giving bath or changing linen, tuck tent under pillow to conserve oxygen.
• Prevent patient from feeling isolated by talking to him. Use a normal tone; the tent doesn't impair hearing.

VENTURI MASK

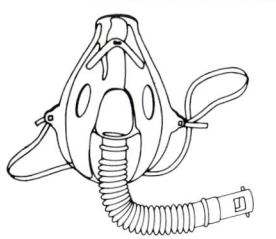

(High-flow system)
Benefits
• Delivers exact oxygen concentrations despite patient's respiratory pattern
• Diluter jets can be changed, or dial turned, to change oxygen concentration
• Doesn't dry mucous membranes
• Can be used to deliver humidity or aerosol therapy
• Never delivers more than the prescribed oxygen concentration.
Problems to expect
• Hot and confining; mask may irritate skin
• FIO_2 may be altered if mask doesn't fit snugly, if tubing's kinked, if oxygen intake ports are blocked, or if less than recommended liter flow is used
• Interferes with eating and talking
• Condensation may collect and drain on patient if humidification is being used.
To avoid complications
• Check ABGs frequently.
• Soften skin around mouth with petrolatum jelly.
• Remove and clean mask every 8 hours with a wet cloth.

Oxygen Therapy Danger Signs

Respiratory depression

When a patient has COPD, hypoxemia becomes his main stimulus to breathe. If you give him too much oxygen, you may remove that stimulus and cause apnea. Prevent it by watching for these danger signs: somnolence and decreased respiration rate. Avoid giving high concentrations of oxygen. Make sure you have an ambubag handy in case of emergency.

Circulatory depression

When a patient has COPD, hypoxemia can cause vasoconstriction. Oxygen therapy reverses this condition and dilates the blood vessels. It may also cause a serious drop in the patient's blood pressure. Prevent this by taking frequent CVP readings and monitoring his blood pressure for changes.

Atelectasis

When a patient receives a high oxygen concentration, the oxygen is exchanged, and the remaining nitrogen is washed from his lungs. This can lead to atelectasis. Do your best to prevent it by making sure your patient coughs and deep breathes on schedule. Hyperinflate his lungs, if necessary.

Oxygen toxicity.

When a patient receives a high oxygen concentration for a prolonged period, serious lung damage or blindness (in newborn infants) can occur. To prevent this, intervene to improve patient's ventilation with chest physiotherapy and suctioning. Monitor blood gas measurements for signs of improvement.

GIVING OXYGEN

Assessing the Effects of Oxygen Use

If your patient will be using oxygen at home, he and his family need to know when he's not getting enough oxygen and when he's getting too much.

Teach them to recognize the signs and symptoms of hypoxemia, which include air hunger (fast, labored breathing), apprehension, change in patient's normal skin color, restlessness, and confusion. Warn the patient or family to notify the doctor at once (or call a local emergency service if he can't reach the doctor immediately) if he experiences any of these symptoms. Your patient may be tempted to increase the flow rate if he feels he's not getting enough oxygen. However, he should never change the oxygen flow rate, unless the doctor orders.

Note: If you're checking on a patient at home, and notice that he's changed the flow rate, find out why he's done so. Discourage him strongly from doing it again. If he feel's he's not receiving enough oxygen, or is having some other difficulty, contact the doctor immediately. If he continues to change the flow rate, suggest that the family obtain a locking flow meter.

Receiving *too much* oxygen can be a problem for your geriatric patient because many older people have age-related respiratory changes. This prevents normal oxygen diffusion into the blood, causing decreased PaO_2. When this happens, low oxygen levels replace high carbon dioxide levels as a respiratory stimulus. If your patient receives too much oxygen, he could develop carbon dioxide narcosis. Signs and symptoms include headache, lethargy, slurred speech, difficulty being aroused, reduced respiratory rate, shallow breathing, coma, and apnea. He or his family should notify the doctor or other emergency assistance immediately.

GIVING OXYGEN

Reducing Oxygen Hazards

A high oxygen concentration will make a fire burn hotter and more rapidly. And, it can make smoldering objects, such as cigarettes, burst into flame. Also, oxygen under pressure may explode when subjected to heat. To help protect your patient and his family from these hazards, give them the following safety instructions:
• Notify the local fire department that oxygen is in the house.
• Keep the oxygen source (usually a tank or concentrator) at least 5′ (1.5 m) from a heat source. If the patient's confined to bed and the heat source is stationary (for example, a radiator or baseboard heater), turn it off, if possible, and place an alternate heat source at a safe distance from the oxygen. *Never* use a fireplace for heat.
• Take stringent measures to prevent smoking. Post large, clearly printed *No smoking* signs on the front door of the house and on the door of the patient's room, as well as inside his room. Doing so will alert visitors not to smoke. Also, make sure they don't give the patient any smoking materials or matches.
• Avoid creating static electricity during oxygen use by having the patient wear all cotton (or at least 85% cotton and 15% synthetic fabric) and use all cotton sheets and blankets, if possible.

• Keep electrical devices at least 5′ (1.5 m) away from the oxygen. Use a straight razor instead of an electrical razor when shaving during oxygen use. Avoid electric heating pads and electric blankets.
• Remove all candles from the patient's room. Give him a flashlight to keep in case of power failure, or if a light bulb burns out.
• Keep all aerosol cans out of the patient's room.
• Prohibit use of lotions, creams, or other products with oil or alcohol during oxygen use and for 3 to 6 hours after use is stopped. Alcohol and oil are both flammable. And, oxygen remains in linens and clothing for as long as 3 to 6 hours after use. Substitute glycerin when giving body rubs. Instead of a temperature-reducing alcohol bath, use ice bags or towels moistened with cool water.
• Keep the patient's hands oil- and grease-free.
• Don't use petroleum jelly or other oil-based moisturizers to relieve facial dryness. Use water-soluble lubricating jelly instead.
• Never lubricate any oxygen delivery equipment.
• Keep a fire extinguisher on hand. Make sure the patient and his family know how to use it.
• Apply these rules when using *portable* oxygen equipment as well as stationary equipment.

Using Liquid Oxygen Safely

Teach your patient the following safety measures for liquid oxygen:
• Keep oxygen supply valves turned off when equipment's not in use.
• Always keep the portable Walker unit and reservoir units upright. Never lay them on their sides.
• Keep the Walker and reservoir in a well-ventilated area (rather than in a drawer, cupboard, or closet), because they continually vent a small flow of pure oxygen through their pressure-relief valves. Confining them in a small space may create an oxygen-rich atmosphere. For the same reason, never carry the Walker under your coat or other clothing.
• Don't run oxygen tubing under your clothing, bed covers, furniture, or carpets.
• In a car, always keep windows or vents open for adequate ventilation; never place the oxygen container in the trunk.
  Note: Consult the supplier for information on traveling with the Walker.
• If you must move the reservoir, handle it carefully. Always lift it with two hands. Don't tip it or try to roll or walk it.
• Hold the Walker by its shoulder strap. Never lift it by the hose or by the hinged cover.
• Because liquid oxygen's so cold, piping and other metal parts can cause frostbite injury on contact, especially during filling. Never touch frosted fittings or piping with your bare hands. Be particularly careful if you have a circulatory problem.
• Warn the patient to consult the supplier if the oxygen gas coming from the cannula feels uncomfortably cool.
• Open doors and windows to ventilate the room while you're filling the Walker. If liquid or cold gas escapes from the fill couplers, stand clear of it, and call the service representative immediately.
• Have the service representative maintain the units regularly. Follow his instructions for connecting breathing equipment, dealing with condensation problems, and filling the Walker from the reservoir.
• Contact the supplier immediately in case of an emergency. Remember to keep his phone number taped to your telephone.
• Use only warm water and household detergent for cleaning the Walker. Don't use alcohol, solvents, polishes, or any oily substances on the Walker or reservoir. Never try to sterilize the Walker or the reservoir.
• Keep oxygen equipment out of the reach of unsupervised children.
• Caution the patient never to increase the liter flow above the prescribed rate.

GIVING OXYGEN

Guide to Humidifiers and Nebulizers

COLD BUBBLE

Advantages
• Can be used with all oxy-gen masks, nasal cannulas, and nasal catheters.
Disadvantages
• Delivers only 20% to 40% humidity
• Can't be used on patient with bypassed upper airway; for example, a tracheostomy.
To avoid complications
• Replace humidifier, or refill it, as water evaporates. *Important:* Always empty the jar completely; then refill it to the proper level.
• If it's not disposable, steril-ize humidifier before using it for another patient.

CASCADE, OR BUBBLE, HUMIDIFIER (heated)

Advantages
• Delivers 100% humidity at body temperature
• Functions as mainstream humidifier with ventilator
• Most effective of all evapo-rative humidifiers.

Disadvantages
• Temperature control can become defective from con-stant use, causing device to overheat or underheat.
• If correct water level isn't maintained, patient's mucosa can become irritated from breathing hot, dry air.
To avoid complications
• Check cascade tempera-ture every 2 hours. Don't let it exceed 101.6° F. (38.6° C.).
• Check the water level at least once every 4 hours. When you add water, empty the reservoir completely; then refill to correct level.
• Attach reservoir tightly.
• If humidifier is overheated, unplug it and let it cool. At-tach another cascade to con-tinue humidification of the patient.

PNEUMATIC (JET) RESER-VOIR NEBULIZER (heated or cool)

Advantages
• Heated nebulizer provides 100% humidity; cool nebu-lizer provides 40% humidity.

Continued

GIVING OXYGEN

Guide to Humidifiers and Nebulizers
Continued

PNEUMATIC (JET) RESER-
VOIR NEBULIZER
Continued

• Useful for long-term therapy
• Can provide both oxygen
and aerosol therapy
• Attaches to wall unit or cyl-
inders.
Disadvantages
• Nondisposable units in-
crease risk of bacterial
growth.
• Condensation can collect in
wide-bore tubing.
• If correct water level in reservoir isn't maintained, patient's mucosa can become
irritated from breathing hot,
dry air.
• Infant can easily become
overhydrated from mist.
To avoid complications
• If patient's upper airway is
bypassed, use a heated nebulizer.
• Check water level in reservoir at least once every 4
hours. When you add water,
empty the reservoir com-
pletely; then refill to correct
level.
• Drain condensation from

wide-bore tubing as soon as
it collects. Don't drain water
back into reservoir.
• Make sure the nebulizer's always delivering a visible mist.
• Weigh infant daily. Watch for
signs of overhydration: weight
gain, pulmonary edema, rales,
electrolyte imbalance.

MOLECULAR HUMIDIFIER
(heated)

Advantages
• Delivers 100% humidity at
body temperature
• Disposable, except for
heating element
• Newer kinds are totally disposable.
Disadvantages
• Same as for cascade hu-
midifier
• Infant can easily become
overhydrated from mist.
To avoid complications
• Observe same precautions
listed for cascade humidifier.
• Change tubing filters every
time you change tubing. Don't
use same filter for more than
one patient.

Continued

GIVING OXYGEN

Guide to Humidifiers and Nebulizers
Continued

MOLECULAR HUMIDIFIER
Continued

• Check mist temperature near infant's mouth. Don't let it exceed 95° F. (35° C.) because humidification will be too great.
• Weigh infant daily. Watch for signs of overhydration: weight gain, pulmonary edema, rales, electrolyte imbalance.

METERED-DOSE NEBULIZER

Advantages
• Effectively delivers bronchodilator; each spray delivers a measured amount of medication.
Disadvantages
• Difficult to assemble
• Patient may use it excessively, because it's available without a prescription.
To avoid complications
• Instruct patient how to use nebulizer.
• Make sure patient doesn't exceed prescribed daily dosage.

• Put mouthpiece and cap on nebulizer after each use to prevent contamination.

ULTRASONIC NEBULIZER

Advantages
• Delivers 100% humidity
• About 90% of the particles will reach the lower airways, where they're effective.
• Loosens secretions.
Disadvantages
• May precipitate bronchospasms in patient with asthma
• Lacks built-in oxygen delivery system
• Increased water absorption may cause overhydration, leading to pulmonary edema or increased cardiac work load.
To avoid complications
• Closely observe patient during and immediately after therapy. His secretions may be so copious and thin that you'll have to assist him.
• Watch for signs of overhydration: weight gain, pulmonary edema, crackles, electrolyte imbalance.

Continued

GIVING OXYGEN

Guide to Humidifiers and Nebulizers
Continued

MAXI-MIST OR MINI-NEBU-
LIZER

Advantages
● Conforms to patient's physiology, allowing him to inhale and exhale with his own power
● Causes less air trapping than IPPB
● Can be used with compressed air, oxygen, or compressor pump
● Compact, disposable unit.
Disadvantages
● Procedure can take a long time if patient requires the nurse's assistance. Patient must be alert and cooperative. Medication may not distribute evenly if patient doesn't breathe properly.
To avoid complications
● Instruct the patient to breathe slowly and deeply. Take time to coach the weak or elderly patient. Assist by holding the apparatus, when necessary.
● Instruct the patient to keep the medicine cup upright during treatment.

● Make sure tubing connections are tight; check for a good mist.

INTERMITTENT POSITIVE
PRESSURE BREATHING
(IPPB)

Advantages
● Mechanically dilates bronchi and lungs; delivers bronchodilator to patient who can't generate an adequate tidal volume
● May prevent atelectasis
● Counteracts pulmonary congestion or edema; helps clear bronchial secretions
● Can give treatment with oxygen or compressed air, depending on doctor's order.
Disadvantages
● Delivers only 40% to 50% oxygen
● Some COPD patients can't tolerate IPPB treatments with oxygen; when this happens, use compressed air.
● May decrease venous return.

GIVING OXYGEN

Continued

Guide to Humidifiers and Nebulizers
Continued

INTERMITTENT POSITIVE
PRESSURE BREATHING
(IPPB) *Continued*

To avoid complications
● Encourage patient to take
slow, deep breaths. Don't allow him to become tachyp-
neic.
● Avoid excess pressures and
high flow rates. Monitor pulse
rates before, during, and after
treatment. Sudden increase
could indicate reaction to
bronchodilator.
● Watch COPD patients for
signs of carbon dioxide nar-

cosis: for example, lethargy
and decreased respiratory
rate.
● Patients with cardiac or pulmonary deficiencies may develop decreased venous
return.
● Don't use in patients with
hemoptysis, pneumothorax,
active TB, or subcutaneous
emphysema.
● Don't use immediately
postop pneumonectomy or lo-
bectomy.
● Don't overdo treatments
with saline solution, because
they're not as effective as
previously believed.

GIVING OXYGEN

Special Consideration

Tell the patient who is using a room humidifier at home that he can fill it
with plain tap water, but that he should periodically run the unit with distilled water *to dissolve the mineral deposits left by the tap water.* To
clean the humidifier, instruct him to run the unit occasionally with a solution of chlorine bleach and distilled water in the reservoir. This should
be done in a well-ventilated room every 5 days *to prevent the otherwise
rapid accumulation of mold and bacteria.*

   Check thermometer readings regularly. Constant use, flow rates below 1 to 4 liters/minute, and insufficient water in the humidifier can
cause the heating device to overheat, raising the temperature of the inspired gas. While water in a heated humidifier may reach temperatures
up to 140° F. (60° C.), it cools as it passes through the tubing, and
should be close to body temperature as the patient breathes it. A range
of 90° to 100° F. (32.2° to 37.8° C.) is acceptable.

Understanding Chest Physiotherapy

You can use chest physiotherapy techniques to prevent or relieve respiratory problems. For example, the doctor may order it if your patient's on prolonged bed rest, or if he's developed atelectasis or pneumonia.

The three techniques described here are most effective when performed together. Explain the procedure to the patient and his family before you begin.

POSTURAL DRAINAGE

Purpose

Postural drainage enables pulmonary secretions to drain by gravity into the major bronchi or the trachea. Then, your patient can dislodge them by coughing. If he can't, he may need percussion and/or vibration techniques.

Procedure

• Place the lung segment to be drained uppermost, with the mainstem bronchus as close to vertical as possible. Remember, positions for postural drainage vary, depending on which lung segment's involved.

Nursing considerations

• Don't perform postural drainage immediately after the patient eats.
• When you drain lower lobes, decrease the drainage angle if your patient can't tolerate the necessary angle (for example, if he has chronic obstructive pulmonary disease).
• Don't use Trendelenburg's position if your patient has increased intracranial pressure or acute heart disease, or has had major abdominal or brain surgery.
• Monitor your patient's cardiac and respiratory status during treatment.

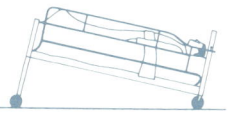

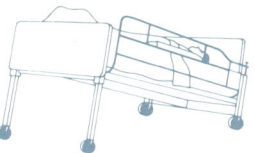

Continued

Understanding Chest Physiotherapy
Continued

PERCUSSION

Purpose
Percussion mechanically dislodges thick, tenacious secretions from the bronchial walls so they can be expectorated or suctioned.

Procedure
• Hold your hands in a cupped shape. Keep your fingers flexed and your thumb tight against your index finger.
• Percuss the chest segment you're draining by alternating your hands in a rhythmic manner. For the technique to work effectively, you must trap air between your hand and the patient's chest. You should hear a hollow sound when doing the procedure—not a loud slap.

Nursing considerations
• Always have a towel, sheet, or patient gown between your hands and the patient's skin. Percuss for 3 to 5 minutes while your patient's in each postural drainage position.

• Don't percuss over your patient's spine or sternum, or below his thoracic cage.
• Avoid percussion if your patient has rib or spinal fractures, flail chest or other traumatic chest injury, pulmonary hemorrhage, pulmonary embolus, mastectomy with silicone implant, metastatic lesion of ribs, pneumothorax, or hemothorax.

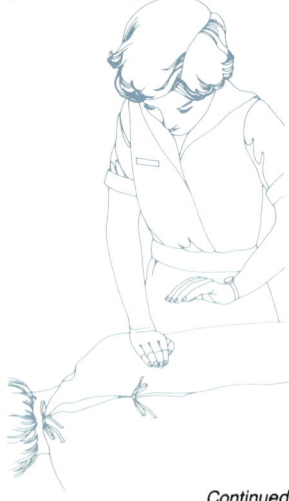

Continued

Understanding Chest Physiotherapy
Continued

VIBRATION

Purpose
Vibration increases velocity and turbulence of exhaled air. This loosens secretions and helps propel them into the larger bronchi so they can be expectorated or suctioned.

Procedure
• Place your hands flat (side by side with your fingers extended) on the chest segment you're draining.
• Instruct your patient to inhale deeply. Then, as he *slowly* exhales, vibrate his chest by quickly contracting and relaxing the muscles of your arms and shoulders. Stop vibrating when he inhales again. Repeat this procedure several times.

Nursing considerations
• Use vibration instead of percussion if your patient has extreme pain in chest area, is frail, or has just had thoracic surgery.
• Vibrate your patient's chest in each postural drainage position. If the doctor orders, alternate this method with percussion.
• Don't vibrate over your patient's spine or sternum, or below his thoracic cage.
• Avoid pressing hard on the patient's ribs, since this may be painful.
• Try to synchronize vibrations with patient's exhalations.
Nursing tip: Consider using a specially-designed electric vibrator (if available) to produce the same effect.

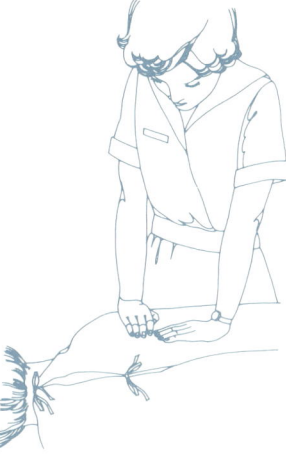

Positioning Patients for Bronchial Drainage

To drain *the posterior basal segments of the lower lobes,* elevate the foot of the table 18″ (45 cm), or 30°, or change the elevation of the foot of the bed to simulate the table. Instruct the patient to lie on his abdomen with his head lowered. Then, position pillows as shown here. Percuss his lower ribs on both sides of his spine.

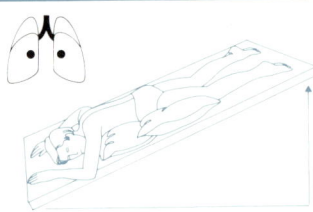

To drain *the lateral basal segments of the lower lobes,* elevate the foot of the table 18″ (45 cm), or 30°. Instruct the patient to lie on his abdomen with his head lowered and his upper leg flexed over a pillow for support. Then have him rotate a quarter turn upward. Percuss his lower ribs on the uppermost portion of his lateral chest wall.

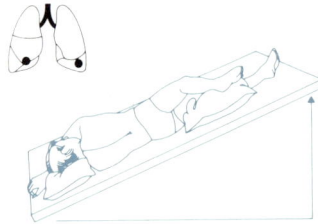

To drain *the anterior basal segments of the lower lobes,* elevate the foot of the table 18″ (45 cm), or 30°. Instruct the patient to lie on his side with his head lowered. Then, place pillows as shown here. Percuss with a slightly cupped hand over his lower ribs just beneath the axilla. *Note:* If an acutely ill patient experiences breathing difficulty in this position, adjust the angle of the bed or table to one he can tolerate. Then, begin percussion.

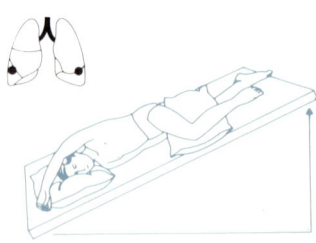

Continued

Positioning Patients for Bronchial Drainage
Continued

To drain *the superior segments of the lower lobes,* make sure the table is flat. Instruct the patient to lie on his abdomen, and place two pillows under his hips. Percuss on both sides of his spine at the lower tip of his scapulae.

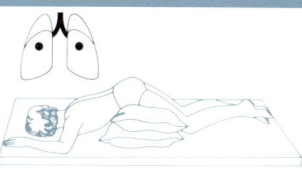

To drain *the medial and lateral segments of the right middle lobe,* elevate the foot of the table 14″ (35 cm), or 15°. Have the patient lie on the left side with his head lowered and his knees flexed, then rotate him a quarter turn backward. Place a pillow beneath him, as shown here. Percuss with your hand moderately cupped over the right nipple. In females, cup your hand so its heel is under the armpit and your fingers extend forward beneath the patient's breast.

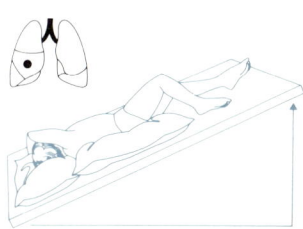

To drain *the superior and inferior segments of the lingular portion of the left upper lobe,* elevate the foot of the table 14″ (35 cm), or 15°. Have the patient lie on his right side with head lowered and knees flexed. Then have him rotate a quarter turn backward. Place a pillow behind him, from shoulders to hips. Percuss with your hand moderately cupped over his left nipple. In females, cup your hand as described above.

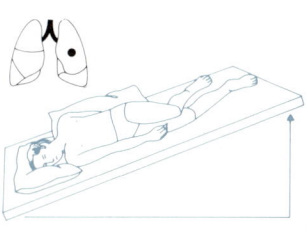

Continued

PROVIDING VENTILATION

Positioning Patients for Bronchial Drainage
Continued

To drain *the anterior segments of the upper lobes,* make sure the table is flat. Instruct the patient to lie on his back with a pillow folded under his knees. Then, have him rotate slightly away from the side being drained. Percuss between his clavicle and nipple.

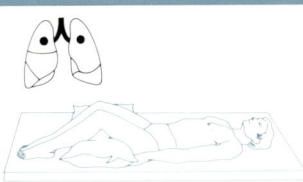

To drain *the apical segment of the right upper lobe and the apical subsegment of the apical-posterior segment of the left upper lobe,* keep the table flat. Have the patient lean back on a pillow at a 30° angle against you. Percuss with your hand cupped between his clavicle and the top of each scapula.

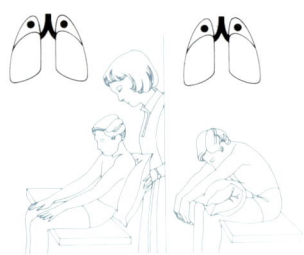

To drain *the posterior segment of the right upper lobe and the posterior subsegment of the apical-posterior segment of the left upper lobe,* keep the table flat. Have the patient lean over folded pillow at 30° angle. Stand behind him; percuss and clap his upper back on each side.

Comparing Ventilators

Ventilators come in two main types—volume-cycled and pressure-cycled—which end inspiration after delivery of a preset volume or pressure. A third ventilator type is time-cycled, meaning it ends inspiration after a preset time has elapsed. (The high-frequency jet ventilator's an example.) Use the chart below to compare ventilators.

VOLUME-CYCLED VENTILATOR

Features
• Ventilator delivers preset tidal volume to lungs.
• Inspiration ends with preset volume delivery.
• Amount of pressure delivered varies with patient's lung compliance.
• Preset volume determines inspiration depth.
• Pop-off safety valve releases pressure when high pressure's required to deliver preset volume.
• Oxygen concentration can be varied between 21% and 100% by changing oxygen flow rate.
• Automatic sigh mechanism helps prevent atelectasis.
• Alarms indicate problems with volume and pressure delivery and sensitivity.
• Electricity powers ventilator.
Indications
• Long-term ventilation
• Severe bronchospasm or adult respiratory distress syndrome (ARDS), which require inflation pressures greater than 40 cmH_2O
• Flail chest, when stabilization requires adequate lung expansion

• Pulmonary edema with decreased compliance
• Cardiac or respiratory arrest
• Central nervous system (CNS) and musculoskeletal disorders (for example, Guillain-Barré syndrome)
• Complex thoracic surgery
• Exacerbated chronic lung disease
• Crushed chest injuries
• PEEP therapy
Advantages
• Changes in airway resistance or compliance have little effect on volume delivered.
• Ventilator delivers precise oxygen concentration.
• Ventilator provides automatic sighing.
Disadvantages
None

PRESSURE-CYCLED VENTILATOR

Features
• Ventilator delivers preset pressure to patient's lungs.
• Inspiration ends with preset pressure delivery.
• Volume of air delivered varies with patient's lung compliance.

Continued

PROVIDING VENTILATION

Comparing Ventilators
Continued

PRESSURE-CYCLED
VENTILATOR
Continued

• Preset pressure determines inspiration depth.
• Air-mix dial delivers oxygen concentration between 40% and 90%; wall outlet delivers 100% oxygen; compressed air from wall outlet delivers 21% oxygen; blenders of compressed air and oxygen deliver oxygen concentrations ranging from 21% to 90%.
• Sigh mechanism operates manually.
• Oxygen or compressed air powers ventilator.
Indications
• Short-term ventilation
• Neuromuscular disease such as myasthenia gravis
• Neurologic disorders that damage respiratory centers in the brain but don't affect lungs
• Intermittent positive pressure breathing (IPPB) therapy
Advantages
• Pressure cycling may ventilate obstructed air passages more efficiently than volume cycling.
Disadvantages
• Older models have limited flow-rate and inspiratory pressure operations.
• Rapid cycling, caused by a kink in tubing or an obstruction, often occurs.

• Continuation of inspiratory phase (a malfunction caused by leaks or electrical disconnection) often occurs.
• A decrease in lung compliance requires a pressure adjustment to maintain alveolar ventilation.
• Routine care, such as turning and suctioning, and coughing and deep-breathing exercises may reduce tidal volume.
• The pressure-cycled ventilator may not deliver the minute volume necessary for long-term mechanical ventilation, since lung compliance changes can alter the tidal volume delivered.

TIME-CYCLED VENTILATOR
(high-frequency jet ventilator)

Features
• Ventilator delivers 100 to 600 breaths/minute with low tidal volume under considerable pressure.
• Jet flow transfers kinetic energy to gases in upper airway moving in the direction of jet flow.
• Inspiration ends after a preset timing cycle has elapsed.
• Timer allows selection of respiratory rate and inspiratory/ expiratory pressure.
• Jet mixing supplies air and oxygen at a pressure of 50 psi.
• Alarm sounds when system malfunctions.

Continued

Comparing Ventilators
Continued

TIME-CYCLED VENTILATOR
Continued

• Driving pressure determines tidal volume.
Indications
• Bronchopleural fistula
• Tracheoesophageal fistula
• Barotrauma, such as pneumothorax and pneumomediastinum
• Low pulmonary compliance (experimentally)
• ARDS (experimentally)
• PEEP therapy (experimentally)
• Flail chest or thoracic trauma

Advantages
• May decrease time required on ventilator and shorten weaning period
• Achieves alveolar ventilation without generating high-peak inspiratory pressure
• Prevents loss of tidal volume through airway disruption site by delivering constant pressure
• Provides lower CO_2 clearance and higher $Paco_2$
• Decreases risk of barotrauma
Disadvantages
• Long-term effects unknown

Phrenic Pacing: A Ventilatory Alternative

The phrenic, or diaphragm, pacemaker helps the patient breathe by stimulating the phrenic nerve. It keeps some patients from long-term dependence on a mechanical ventilator.

A diaphragm pacemaker is usually attached to the left phrenic nerve. Any damage that may occur there will affect pulmonary function less than damage to the right phrenic nerve, which controls ventilation of the larger right lung.

A single pacemaker's usually enough for the patient who has a disease that allows him to breathe on his own while awake. But for the patient who can't, two pacemakers, each one used for no more than 12 hours at a time, may prevent fatigue.

To insert the pacemaker, the doctor surgically implants an electrode around the phrenic nerve where it crosses the scalenus anticus muscle. Then, he attaches the electrode to a separate subcutaneous receiver.

Once the patient's phrenic nerve's activated, his diaphragm will move. Here's how: A current flows from the transmitter to the antenna, then to the receiver through the electrode connectors, and then to the electrode cuff.

Coping with Mechanical Ventilation Complications

BAROTRAUMA

Takes the form of pneumothorax, subcutaneous emphysema, or mediastinal emphysema; usually caused when volume and pressure settings are too high or during administration of PEEP

Signs and symptoms

Sudden cyanosis; sudden drop in blood pressure; sudden decrease in lung compliance; increased anxiety. With pneumothorax, patient may have absent or diminished breath sounds over affected lung segment, acute pain on affected side, and trachea deviated away from pneumothorax. With subcutaneous emphysema, patient may have crepitus of face, abdomen, and extremities. With mediastinal emphysema, patient shows signs of reduced cardiac output and of crepitus over heart area.

Intervention

• Call doctor immediately; he may insert chest tubes.

Prevention

• Avoid high-pressure settings for high-risk patients; for example, those with chronic obstructive pulmonary disease (COPD), emphysematous blebs, or pulmonary scar tissue.

ATELECTASIS

Caused by insufficient deep breathing, pneumothorax, secretion retention, or a combination of these

Signs and symptoms

Transient fine crackles; diminished breath sounds over affected lung segment; bronchial sounds over peripheral lung fields; decreased compliance; possible change in arterial blood gas (ABG) values

Intervention

• Turn patient frequently.
• Suction and hyperinflate patient's lungs periodically.
• Use intermittent sighing.
• Perform chest physiotherapy, as ordered.
• Doctor may order bronchoscopy.

Prevention

• Change patient's position every 1 to 2 hours and maintain good body alignment.
• Give chest physiotherapy, and maintain good pulmonary hygiene.
• Doctor may order PEEP.
• Suction the patient, as needed.
• Remember to sigh patient frequently.
• Monitor the patient closely.

Continued

Coping with Mechanical Ventilation Complications
Continued

CARDIOVASCULAR IMPAIRMENT

Caused when positive intrathoracic pressure reduces venous return to heart's right side and compresses pulmonary blood circulation

Signs and symptoms
Decreased blood pressure and cardiac output; possible decreased urinary output; increased central venous pressure and pulmonary artery pressure; increased heart rate

Intervention
• Doctor may reduce intrathoracic pressure by decreasing PEEP, inspiratory flow rate, or tidal volume.
• Doctor may order increased I.V. fluids or administration of plasma expanders such as albumin or colloidal substances.

Prevention
• Monitor Pao$_2$ closely. It should not fall below 70 mm Hg.
• Use PEEP only when necessary.
• Shorten inspiration time to less than one half expiration time.
• Maintain adequate blood volume.

GASTROINTESTINAL COMPLICATIONS (GI bleeding, gastric distention, paralytic ileus, and stress ulcer)

Caused by stress or swallowing air

Signs and symptoms
Abdominal distention; steady decrease in hemoglobin and hematocrit measurement; positive hematest results on nasogastric drainage and stool; tarry stool

Intervention
• As ordered, insert nasogastric tube for drainage.
• Replace lost blood.
• Use nasogastric tube to give antacids or other medication to decrease acid production.

Prevention
• Avoid giving excessive positive pressure.
• Reduce patient's psychological stress.
• Give antacids and other medications to reduce acid production, as ordered.

ACID-BASE AND FLUID AND ELECTROLYTE IMBALANCE

Caused by positive water balance created by secretion of antidiuretic hormone (ADH); also caused by reduced insensible losses from respiratory tract

Continued

Coping with Mechanical Ventilation Complications
Continued

ACID-BASE AND FLUID AND
ELECTROLYTE IMBALANCE
Continued

Signs and symptoms
Probable change in blood gas
measurements; decreased vital
capacity; weight gain; ankle
edema; moist crackles in lungs'
lower lobes; pulmonary edema
confirmed by X-ray
Intervention
• Doctor may restrict fluid intake
and order diuretics.
• Take nursing measures for congestive heart failure (CHF), as ordered.
• Apply rotating tourniquets to
control pulmonary edema, as ordered.
• Correct acid-base and electrolyte imbalance, as ordered.
Prevention
• Periodically obtain blood samples
for ABG and electrolyte measurements. Monitor patient for hyperventilation or hypoventilation.
• Monitor patient's fluid intake and
output.
• Weigh patient daily.

TRACHEAL TRAUMA

Caused by constant pressure of
cuffed endotracheal tube or nasal
endotracheal tube on the patient's
trachea

Signs and symptoms
Decreased tidal volume from air
leak; bleeding from trachea
Intervention
• Depending on damage, the doctor may insert a new trach tube to
change cuff's position and allow
injured area to heal.
• Give meticulous cuff care, using
minimal leak technique, until tube
can be removed.
Prevention
• Give patient proper cuff care,
using minimal leak technique
when possible.
• Doctor should use endotracheal
or trach tubes with soft cuffs.

RESPIRATORY INFECTION

Caused when upper airway is bypassed, eliminating body's natural
defense mechanisms against infection; also caused by poor
aseptic technique
Signs and symptoms
Elevated temperature and white
blood cell count (WBC); increased
amount of respiratory secretions,
and change in their color and
odor
Intervention
• Notify doctor.
• Change patient's position frequently and perform chest physiotherapy.
• Use aseptic technique for trach
care and for suctioning.

Continued

PROVIDING VENTILATION

Coping with Mechanical Ventilation Complications
Continued

RESPIRATORY INFECTION
Continued

• Administer prescribed antibiotics.
Prevention
• Maintain good pulmonary hygiene by using aseptic technique and sterile equipment, changing ventilator tubing every 24 hours, and suctioning patient and hyperinflating his lungs as needed.
• Turn patient frequently.
• Perform chest physiotherapy.
• Filter all inspired gas.

OXYGEN TOXICITY

Caused by excessively high concentrations of oxygen (over 60%) administered over prolonged period (8 hours or more); may cause fibrotic tissue changes in lungs, possibly leading to death

Signs and symptoms
Retrosternal pain; sore throat; nasal congestion; burning chest pain on inspiration; dry, hacking cough; dyspnea; decreased compliance; decreased PaO_2 on the same oxygen concentration; decreased vital capacity; and X-ray changes
Intervention
• Monitor oxygen levels carefully. Report signs of oxygen toxicosis immediately.
Prevention
• Maintain good pulmonary hygiene so low oxygen concentrations are adequate.
• Reduce oxygen concentrations as soon as possible.
• Use PEEP to reduce oxygen concentration level, as ordered.

Nursing Tip

If your patient's receiving a neuromuscular blocking drug like Pavulon while on a ventilator, his eyes won't blink or tear. Keep them moist by instilling prescribed eyedrops or washing them with sterile saline solution. To protect them further, close his eyelids and cover them with ¼" nonallergenic tape or oval eye patches.

Troubleshooting the TcpO₂ Monitor

The transcutaneous oxygen (TcpO₂) monitor, which monitors blood oxygen tension noninvasively, is painless for the patient and simple to operate. If the patient's oxygen tension measurement, detected by body sensors, falls below or rises above the set limit, an alarm will sound.

Read this chart to learn about TcpO₂ monitoring problems. You'll see what may cause them and find out how to deal with them.

POWER LIGHT DOESN'T LIGHT

Possible causes
• Unplugged monitor
• Disconnected sensor cable
• Defective sensor cable
• Faulty wall outlet
• Monitor fuse blown
Nursing action
• Plug monitor into wall outlet.
• Secure connections at both ends of the sensor cable.
• Replace sensor cable.
• Use a different wall outlet.
• Consult operator's manual or call for repair service.

TcpO₂ mm Hg DISPLAY IS DARK

Possible cause
• Monitor not warmed up yet
Nursing action
• Allow 10 minutes for the monitor to warm up after you turn on the power.

TREND RECORDER AND HEATER POWER REMAIN AT ZERO

Possible causes
• Disconnected cable between TcpO₂ monitor and trend recorder

Nursing action
• Secure cable connections.

TREND RECORDER CHART READING DOESN'T AGREE WITH PO₂ mm Hg DISPLAY READING ON MONITOR

Possible causes
• Trend recorder paper incorrectly installed
Nursing action
• Refer to operator's manual for proper installation technique.

SENSITIVITY READING IS GREATER THAN 150 mm Hg

Possible causes
• Air bubbles on sensor face, or wrinkled or punctured sensor membrane
Nursing action
• Disassemble and reassemble the sensor.

SENSITIVITY READING IS LESS THAN 50 mm Hg BUT MORE THAN 8 mm Hg

Possible causes
• Too much electrolyte solution under sensor membrane

Continued

Troubleshooting the TcpO₂ Monitor
Continued

SENSITIVITY READING IS LESS
THAN 50 mm Hg BUT MORE
THAN 8 mm Hg *Continued*

- Leaking electrical current
- Faulty sensor membrane
- Deposits on sensor face

Nursing action
- Gently touch the membrane. If
you feel a cushion of liquid, disassemble and reassemble the sensor.
- Check for electrical leakage,
using the procedure described in
your operator's manual.
- Replace membrane.
- Clean sensor with an alcohol
sponge.

SENSITIVITY READING IS LESS
THAN 8 mm Hg

Possible causes
- Sensor completely disconnected
- Sensor malfunctioning
- Monitor malfunctioning

Nursing action
- Carefully reapply sensor at a
different site.
- Call for repair service.

TcpO₂ AND ARTERIAL PaO₂
MEASUREMENTS DON'T CORRELATE

Possible causes
- Air between sensor and skin
- No contact jelly on sensor
- Insufficient thermal stabilization
time
- Sensor temperature too low
- Patient has impaired arterial-alveolar perfusion or other physiologic disturbances, possibly drug-induced.

Nursing action
- Make sure adhesive ring is
tightly sealed. If not, replace it.
- Remove sensor and check it. If
there's no contact jelly on it, correct the problem. Then change
adhesive ring and recalibrate the
sensor to the monitor.
- Allow 5 to 45 minutes for proper
stabilization.
- Increase sensor temperature.
- Remove sensor and reapply it
to another site.
- Notify the doctor. He will order
appropriate treatment.

Special Consideration

Since neonatal skin is very thin, with little subcutaneous fat, TcpO₂,
monitoring is quite accurate. However, in infants with shock or hypoperfusion, results do not accurately reflect arterial values, because blood is
shunted to the heart, brain, and lungs, reducing peripheral blood flow.

PROVIDING VENTILATION

INDEX

INDEX

INDEX

INDEX